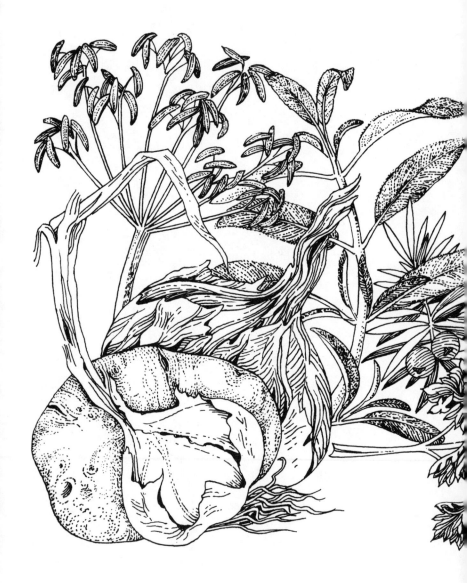

THE BOOK OF HEALTHY FOODS

Vicki Peterson

Illustrated by Yvonne Skargon

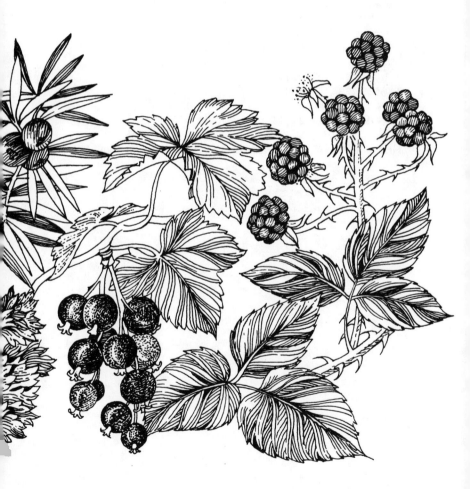

St. Martin's Press/New York

Library of Congress Cataloging in Publication Data

Peterson, Vicki.
   The book of healthy foods.

   1. Food.   2. Nutrition.   I. Title.
TX353.P428   641.5′637   71-5796
ISBN 0-312-08907-4   AACR2
ISBN 0-312-08908-2 (pbk.)

First published in Great Britain by Allen Lane, Penguin Books Ltd.

> CONTENTS <

Contents

> ACKNOWLEDGEMENTS <

Among the many individuals and societies who generously helped me with this book, my thanks are particularly due to the following organizations: the Herb Society, London; the Herb Society of America, Boston; the New York Botanical Gardens, New York; the American Antiquarian Society; the United Society of Shakers; and the International Association of Medical Herbalists, Quebec.

All the information on constituents and nutritive values of foods was taken from details kindly supplied by the Agricultural Research Service of the United States Department of Agriculture.

> INTRODUCTION <

I wrote this book first and foremost because I thought it was high time we had some *good* news about food.

The idea came about, strangely enough, when I was writing another book on natural foods. During the research on the so-called civilized diseases so peculiar to Western countries, I was struck by the doom and gloom we are subjected to these days. By contrast, I began to think of the intuitive wisdom of our not-so-distant ancestors, who could go out into garden or field and select a vegetable, herb or fruit to deal with most of their minor ailments.

At about the same time, I heard of the modern scientific research into onion. Teams of doctors in India and Britain have now established that onion is a fine prevention against heart disease, since it can help the body dissolve the clots which sometimes form inside the blood vessels. This onion research came about because one open-minded Indian doctor, I. S. Menon, did not roar with laughter when a patient chanced to remark that, in France, when a horse develops clots, he is fed a diet of onions and garlic. Dr Menon not only listened, he got together a group of his colleagues and started the series of tests which established onion as a leading food medicine.

Similarly, at Aston University, Dr David Lewis did not dismiss granny's favourite remedy for arthritis, celery seed tea. He began the laboratory tests which were to establish, in his words, that 'celery has a definite anti-inflammatory action'.

From my interest in folk lore I knew that onion is a traditional 'heart strengthener' and that celery is a classic folk remedy for arthritis and rheumatism. I began to think what a good idea it would be somehow to link up these folk uses with modern research. With this glimmer of an idea I spoke to my agent, Peter Grose, who really must be given credit for the whole concept of this book. When I consulted the Herb Society in London, I learned that they had hoped to correlate such research details on a central computer, but lacked the necessary resources. So, with the help of an indefatigable secretary, Jane Little, I wrote 400 letters to doctors and research establishments around the world and consulted computer banks in the U.S.A.

I was mildly astonished when the answers came in. From Warsaw I learned of research into red beetroot; from France findings on olive oil; from the U.S.A. details of the work on cabbage and alcoholism; from Russia the research on cabbage and ginseng. The response from Russia was the most surprising of all. From Professor V. A. Shaternikov at the U.S.S.R. Academy of Medical Sciences in Moscow came a ten-page letter giving details of Russian treatment of peptic ulcers with white cabbage. From the Institute of Biologically Active Substances at Vladivostok I was sent forty pages of fascinating details on ginseng.

From these and other sources I learned that it is official Soviet policy to encourage scientific research into the medicinal activity of vegetables, fruits and herbs. If a natural drug is established, it is used immediately in preference to a synthetic product. For instance, Russian astronauts are given ginseng on their space missions.

It is fair to say, however, that the United States leads the world in general food research. The U.S. Department of Agriculture sponsors detailed research into both the growth and actions of daily food and the way it is absorbed by the body. Throughout the length and breadth of the U.S.A. there is an extraordinary enthusiasm and good will rising from the average man or woman in the street, who is quite prepared to put modern research findings on food straight into the kitchen, and as a writer specializing in food I find this most encouraging.

That the entire American nation did perceptibly alter their national diet as advised by the Government body, the Senate Select Committee, in the late 1970s, was shown in the drop in the rate of heart attacks.

Elsewhere, things are changing slowly but surely. In London supermarkets wholemeal bread often sells out more quickly than white. Ordinary shops sell items which would have been unheard of a few years ago: yogurt, honey, mineral waters, pure fruit juices, olive oil. Around the world, Australians have taken to herb teas and mineral waters with their usual vigour. The Europeans have always been conscious that certain foods can help maintain excellent health. The Germans, French, and Italians are used to a superb range of pure, natural juices and medicinal mineral waters. Garlic, onions, beet and yogurt are an important part of their diets.

Other folk uses, too, have come from Europe. The Europeans specialize in the great body 'spring cleaning' rituals once a year in April or May. Certain foods or herbs are selected with great care and knowledge and used as medicaments to speed winter from the system. Often a whole week is spent taking specific vegetable juices or food remedies. These yearly body cleansers have a remarkably stimulating and reinvigorating effect.

Frenchmen, in particular, use their 'spring cures' to renew their physical and mental vitality. Spring is the ideal time for these folk remedies, which I will describe under the various headings which follow. Not only do they speed winter's flu and cold toxins out of the system, they also, to paraphrase Shakespeare, help turn our minds lightly to thoughts of love.

While I was writing this book, I happened to visit Hadrian's Wall in the North East of England. It was a dark, stormy day. The wind was blowing rain in great gusts across the valleys where the conquering legions had marched centuries ago. In the shadow of the great wall stood a cottage, built of the same stone that the Roman soldiers had so laboriously hewn to build their great defensive wall. I was intrigued to see two bulbs of garlic nailed firmly to the cottage door. Knowing this to be the age-old charm to ward off witches and disease, I knocked on the door.

The sprightly old lady who answered might have been forgiven for thinking that her worst fears had been realized, seeing a wet, bedraggled figure standing there. She soon recovered her equanimity and told me of the garlic medicines and spring cures that her family had always used; the pungent garlic unguents and potions, and the May 'reviving' medicine made from garlic, celery and beet juices.

In return, I told her of the folk uses of garlic in France and other lands and she stared at me in astonishment. 'I didn't think the younger generation cared about things like that,' she said.

Also in the North East of England, at Newcastle, I saw a long line of people reaching half-way round the block, queuing to get into a small local shop. It was Sunday morning and I was told that the shopkeeper made an instant hangover cure. The queuers were mostly sailors from visiting international ships, and they presented almost a cartoon picture of the 'morning-after' look – bleary eyes, hands clutched to aching heads. A Norwegian sailor told me, unconsciously echoing Bertie Wooster in P. G. Wodehouse: 'When you swallow this cure, there is a loud explosion in the head, lights before the eyes, then suddenly everything clears.'

I managed to ask the shopkeeper what was in his effective formula. 'It's a family secret, handed down,' he said. Finally, he told me a few of the main ingredients; garlic juice, artichoke elixir, and sarsaparilla. Quite rightly, he refused to divulge the rest of what was a best-selling natural remedy.

The American writer, James Thurber, paints a delightful portrait of natural healing in his book *Alarms and Diversions* (published by Hamish Hamilton). Thurber describes 'Aunt Margery' Albright, who used her considerable natural folk knowledge to save his father from a lingering illness:

I was reminded of Mrs Albright not long ago when I ran across an old query of Emerson's: 'Is it not an eminent convenience to have in your town a person who knows where arnica grows, or sassafras, or pennyroyal?' Mrs Albright was skilled in using the pharmacopoeia of the woods and fields. She could have brought the great philosopher dozens of roots and leaves and barks, good for everything from ache to agony and from pukin' spells to a knotted gut. She could also have found in the countryside around Concord the proper plants for the treatment of asthma and other bronchial disturbances. She gathered belladonna, Jimson weed, and digitalis, made a mixture of them, added a solution of saltpetre, put the stuff in a bowl and set it on fire. The patient simply bent over the bowl and inhaled the fumes. She knew where sour grass grew, which you chew for dyspepsy, and mint, excellent for the naushy, and the slippery elm whose fragrant inner bark was the favorite demulcent of a hundred years ago – the thing to use for raw throat and other sore tishas.

Of course, in urban society, we cannot go into the fields to gather medicinal plants, but we can certainly use our local fruit and vegetable shops as a pharmacopoeia in the light of the facts assembled in this book. Of course, I would prefer you to buy organically grown items to use as remedies if this is at all possible but I realize that this is often hard. For many of us it is easier to grow our own fruit and vegetables than to travel to an organic farm or shop.

Obviously, a book like this takes a good deal of concentrated effort. This was made easier for me by the help of my husband, Bruce Peterson, and my brother, Tim Ashton-Jennings, who did research for me at the Library of Congress, Washington and throughout America.

I have marshalled the facts with care and tried to present them in a readable way, together with some fascinating folk uses and historical legends. Having described all the good things food can do, obviously it seemed a good idea to suggest a few imaginative culinary uses from around the world.

I am not saying for one moment that anyone should attempt self-diagnosis or avoid going to a doctor. What I do believe is that food, correctly chosen, can have a powerful and beneficial effect on your life. I believe that many plants are powerful natural medicines.

The right food ally can help prevent colds, influenza, arthritis and rheumatism and a host of other ailments. With more knowledge about food medicines, you can improve your vitality, virility and resistance to disease.

The re-kindling of our ancient understanding about the medicinally active elements in food has come from the grass roots, in particular, from the people of the U.S.A., Russia and China.

There are signs that more than a few orthodox doctors are responding. A professor of pharmacy described the movement as 'a great tide of green medicine sweeping around the world'.

Changing attitudes to food medicines were neatly summed up by Paul C. Mangelsdorf, former Director of the Botanical Museum at Harvard University. Dr Mangelsdorf said:

When I began to prepare my first lecture on this subject in 1941, I was impressed with what then seemed to be the declining importance of medicinal drugs of plant origin. Of the ten drugs most widely prescribed in the United States at that time, only two – codeine and digitalis – were of plant origin.

... I described this downward trend, told the students that it would undoubtedly continue, and predicted that by the time I would retire some 25 years later medicinal drugs of plant origin would be of little more than historical interest. 27 years have now elapsed since I made this bold prediction, and it turns out that I could scarcely have been more wrong.

Professor Richard Evan Shultes, the distinguished Harvard University ethnobotanist, commented:

Many are the instances where folk uses of plants, had they seriously been followed up, might have led much earlier to valuable discoveries.

What I have tried to do in this book is to give back to you, the reader, some of our traditional wisdom about food learned through centuries of folk uses, and at the same time, link this with modern scientific research.

My hope is that some of this knowledge can go straight into your daily life in the kitchen and help in the common search for vibrant health.

> SELECT BIBLIOGRAPHY <

APICIUS, *The Roman Cookery Book*, a translation by B. Flower and E. Rosenbaum, Harrap, 1958.

CLAUS, E. P., TAYLOR, V. E., and BRADY, L. R., *Pharmacognosy* (6th ed.), Lea & Febiger, Philadelphia, 1970.

DIOSCORIDES, *The Greek Herbal*, Oxford University Press, 1934.

DRUMMOND, J. C., and WILBRAHAM, A., *The Englishman's Food*, Jonathan Cape, 1939.

FERGUSON, N. M., *A Textbook of Pharmacognosy*, Macmillan, New York, 1956.

FLÜCK, HANS, *Medicinal Plants*, translated by J. M. Rowson, W. Foulsham, 1976.

GORDON ROSS, A. C., *Homoeopathic Green Medicine*, Thorsons, 1978.

GRIEVE, MAUDE, *A Modern Herbal*, Penguin Books, 1977.

HARTLEY, DOROTHY, *Food in England*, Macdonald & Jane's, 1954.

KADANS, JOSEPH M., *Encyclopedia of Medicinal Herbs*, Arco, New York, 1972.

KREIG, MARGARET B., *Green Medicine*, Harrap, 1965; Apollo, Chicago, 1971.

LEHNER, E. and J., *Folklore and Odysseys of Food and Medicinal Plants*, Tudor, 1962.

LOEWENFELD, CLAIRE, and BACK, PHILLIPA, *The Complete Book of Herbs and Spices*, David & Charles, 1974; Little, Brown, Boston, 1976.

REVOLUTIONARY HEALTH COMMITTEE OF HUNAN PROVINCE, *A Barefoot Doctor's Manual*, Routledge & Kegan Paul, 1978.

SHARMA, C. H., *A Manual of Homoeopathy and Natural Medicine*, Turnstone Books, 1975.

SWAIN, TONY (ed.), *Plants in the Development of Modern Medicine*, Harvard University Press, 1972.

TAYLOR, N., *Plant Drugs that Changed the World*, Dodd, Mead & Co., New York, 1965.

THOMSON, WILLIAM A. R. (ed.), *Healing Plants: A Modern Herbal*, Macmillan, 1978.

TODD, R. G. (ed.), *Martindale, The Extra Pharmacopoeia* (25th ed.), Pharmaceutical Press, 1967.

TREASE, G. E., and EVANS, W. C., *Pharmacognosy*, (10th ed.), Baillière Tindall, 1972.

USHER, GEORGE, *A Dictionary of Plants Used by Man*, Constable 1974; Hafner Press, New York, 1974.

WREN, R. C., *Potters New Cyclopaedia of Botanical Drugs and Preparations*, Health Science Press, 1956.

⟫ ARTICHOKE ⟪

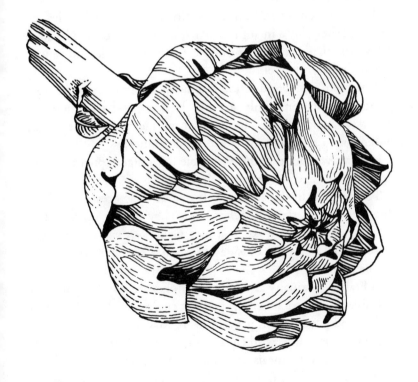

> Health <

The artichoke proper is the globe artichoke, with its tall, elegant stem and prickly thistle-like head. Globe artichoke is closely related to the thistle, and, like all this noble family, possesses excellent therapeutic values.

You might expect a thistle to provide a snag and it is this: to get the major, powerful medicinal effect of this lordly vegetable you should tackle the stem, root and lower leaves as well as the flower head or 'choke'.

By all means go on enjoying the delicious artichoke hearts, since they share the therapeutic values, but be brave and use the rest of the plant as well.

Active substances and other constituents in artichoke's leaves, stem and root play a major role in natural prevention and healing. They stimulate the liver, promote the flow of bile and reduce blood cholesterol levels.

Artichoke's threefold action is unusual and impressive, because plants do not commonly act on the liver and cholesterol in this way. Artichoke also has a vigorous, cleansing effect on the system and a mild diuretic effect on the kidneys.

Is it any wonder that this vegetable has a high reputation both in alternative and folk medicine?

To the French, the artichoke is one of their great 'friends of the liver' and depurative 'cleansers'. They have a saying: 'like the heart of an artichoke' – a nice Gallic *bon mot* describing a person, prickly on the outside but good where it matters most, on the inside.

In France, Germany and Italy artichokes are popularly used to improve poor liver function, prevent cholesterol build-up, treat high blood pressure and prevent heart attacks.

French men and women sipping artichoke aperitifs on the boulevards before meals and watching the world go by in a leisurely way are, in fact, enjoying a sound natural medicine.

> Constituents <

Globe artichoke contains cynarine, enzyme, bitter principle, tannin, mucilage. More of the active constituents are present in the lower leaves, stem and root.

> History <

Artichokes were a popular delicacy at Roman feasts, but Pliny, with one of his occasional lapses of judgement, scolded his contemporaries for paying a lot of money for 'mere thistles'.

Globe artichoke is native to the Mediterranean and North Africa. The word artichoke is a corruption of its Arab name, *al'qarshuf*, indicating that the vegetable was popular in Eastern countries centuries before it was appreciated by the West.

It began to be widely cultivated in France and Britain around the sixteenth century. Parkinson in 1640 referred to the statement by Theophrastus in the fourth century: 'The head of Scolymus is most pleasant, being boyled or eaten raw, but chiefly when it is in flower, as also the inner substance of the heads is eaten.'

The French rapidly became expert in the growing and cooking of artichokes. Tournefort commented in 1730: 'The French and the Germans boil the heads as we do, but the Italians eat them raw with salt and oil and pepper.' A terse statement this, which gave no clue to the infinite variety of Continental artichoke dishes.

> Folk Use <

French people have many ways of making artichoke medicine quite palatable. They steep the root in white wine; the juices are pressed out of the stem and leaves and mixed with madeira or wine, whichever they fancy. The leathery lower leaves are dried for tisanes and then generally mixed with a pleasant-tasting juice such as carrot or celery or simply taken quickly as a medicine on a warm spoon dipped in brandy.

Artichoke elixirs and medicines are taken in France as part of their regular yearly 'cleansing', either in spring or autumn. A more regular dosage is taken by anyone prone to liver troubles.

In Germany and France anyone who frankly enjoys the pleasures of wine takes care to keep his body healthy with one of these traditional aids to the liver.

In the case of artichoke, too, people with rheumatism take regular two- or three-week courses of leaf tisane or root elixir. Folk medicine believes also that artichoke offers good protection against strokes, intestinal viruses and arthritis.

French mothers have passed down from generation to generation the knowledge that artichoke hearts and leaves are good for all the family. This ethnic awareness must contribute to French cuisine's vast and imaginative use of artichoke heads, bottoms and hearts, which offer a food medicine in the nicest possible way.

> **Herbal Medicine** <

Globe artichoke's stimulating effect on the liver makes it a valuable herbal medicine for many disorders of that organ. Artichoke mixtures are most helpful in all liverish or bilious conditions, especially because of the anti-nausea effect. In fact, herbalists treat nausea with a standard brew of artichoke tea made from two teaspoons of artichoke leaves brought to the boil in one cup of water, allowed to stand for 15 minutes, strained and drunk as needed.

Artichoke's other special properties, such as promoting the flow of bile, make it a widely adopted alternative medicine. Herbalists treat gallstones with standard artichoke tea; one cup is taken two or three times a day for four to six weeks.

The other major benefit provided by this excellent vegetable is its cholesterol reducing property, and herbalists put this to good use in many medicines for arterial disease (arteriosclerosis), high blood pressure and certain heart complaints.

> Culinary Use <

In one of his Five Towns novels, Arnold Bennett wove the entire story around the fact that his hero (or anti-hero) Denry was humiliated at a luxury hotel because he did not know how to eat his artichoke. Presented with the thistle-like choke on a platter, Denry attacked it with a spoon, causing a woman fellow diner to hoot with derision. Denry later exacted a terrible revenge on her and thereby hung the whole plot.

There is an art to eating a whole artichoke head gracefully. It is a convivial art, since few Western dishes are served on one plate intended to be shared by several people. (The Chinese are very good at this style of eating.) One artichoke can serve two or three people, depending on the size of the choke and their appetites. Each person has a small plate individually containing an appropriate sauce, such as hollandaise, mousseline, white sauce or simply good hot butter. Everyone gently peels away an artichoke petal, starting at the bottom, and uses it as a scoop to convey the sauce to the mouth, biting off the delicious 'meaty' artichoke bit at the end of the petal at the same time.

Artichokes should be firm, well-coloured and firmly tapering in round a solid centre. To boil them, cut off the stalks, pull off the hard outer leaves, and trim the remaining petals neatly to about two-thirds of their original height. Wash the choke well, tie it with string around the fullest part, then cook it base down in a pan of boiling salted water until the bottom part is tender. The length of time depends on the age and size of the artichoke.

If the chokes are to be served cold, cool them under cold water as soon as they are cooked. Cold boiled artichoke is delicious with mayonnaise, mustard, tartare or vinaigrette.

In French cuisine, artichokes are stuffed with many delicious mixtures, ranging from mushroom, nutmeg and shallot cooked in oil with white wine to common or garden sausage meat.

The most tender and succulent part of the artichoke is the

heart. Young, immature heads are used in Italy, either baked or fried, or eaten raw with a good wine and oil dressing.

Artichoke hearts in brine are canned and exported world-wide from Mediterranean countries, and make excellent additions to pizze, *hors d'oeuvre*, salads and sauces.

> **BEET** <
(beetroot)

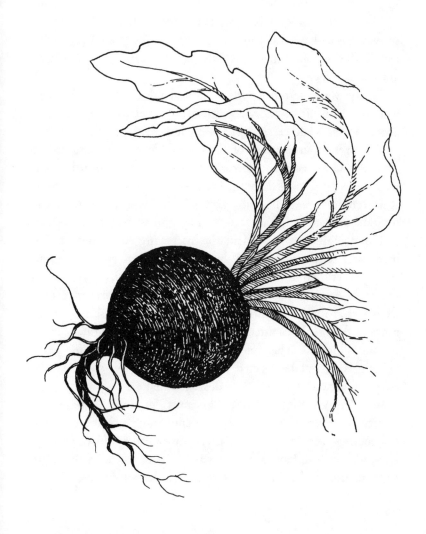

The power of beet as a liver cleanser has been known and made use of by our ancestors for at least eight hundred years. In Eastern Europe, beet juice is also appreciated as a preventative medicine, and used regularly to maintain vibrant health.

In the last decade scientists have analysed beet, but several of the active constituents still remain unidentified, a familiar story in natural medicine. It is known that a major active ingredient in beet is the alkaloid betaine, and research in the U.S.A. has shown this to have a 'significant action' on the liver. Beet is also rich in the enzyme catalese, which is believed to be an important anti-cancer agent.

Today, we have more need of natural aids to liver health than any of our intuitive ancestors. A healthy liver can filter out the array of toxins and carcinogens peculiar to the twentieth century.

The preventative value of this vegetable was investigated at Warsaw University in the early 1970s, where a control group drank raw beet juice daily throughout the three winter months. Researchers found that the group had fewer colds than the national average, and that four overweight members lost weight.

This weight loss is particularly interesting, since beet is rich in natural sugar and usually shunned by slimmers. The clue to the apparent contradiction lies in beet's beneficial action on the liver. An important function of the liver is to prepare fat for transport around the body. Any imbalance can cause symptoms ranging from bilious attacks and fatigue to overweight or more serious illnesses. The researchers concluded that the active principles in red beet acted as a 'trigger' to the complex co-enzymal action in which liver deals with fat.

Beet has yet more to offer. Scientists in England have discovered that beet leaves have oestrogenic or hormonal properties. It becomes clear now why Eastern European women, in their age-old wisdom, have always turned to beet leaf tea to regulate their menses and keep them fertile. The leaves are also rich in iron and provide excellent amounts of vitamin A. In fact, beet leaves are one of the richest natural sources of both iron and vitamin A and contain far more than apricots.

Beet juice taken medicinally in large amounts for short periods can sometimes stain the urine or stool, but do not be alarmed by this.

The anti-cancer activity of beet has been investigated in France and at Helsinki University, but it is too early yet to draw any definite conclusions.

Clearly this vegetable plays an important dual role in the natural foods' armoury against disease. If you use beet regularly your body will be better able to resist colds and infections, and the liver can perform its vital functions most efficiently.

> **Constituents** <

Red beet root contains reasonable amounts of fibre, iron, calcium, potassium, choline, the vitamins A and C and the B vitamins thiamine, riboflavin and niacin.

Beet leaves contain fibre, calcium, potassium, vitamin C and the B vitamins thiamine, riboflavin and niacin, with very rich amounts of iron and vitamin A.

> **History** <

The beet is a native of Southern Europe, where it grows wild in maritime areas of Italy and Greece. It belongs to the same *Chenopodium* family as spinach and Good King Henry, and presents the typical succulent stems of the group which are so ideal for water storage. White beet, *Beta cicla*, is grown mainly for its leaves and is known as chard.

Our botanical name for the vegetable probably comes from the old Celtic word for red – *bett. Vulgaris* indicates that it is in common use, and the family name, *Chenopodium*, refers to the goosefoot shape of the alternate leaves and comes from the Greek *chen*, goose and *pous*, foot.

Red beet was highly prized by the Greeks as a medicinal food, and was introduced by the Roman legions to Britain where it became vastly popular in the form of potent home-made wine. Most country districts still have their traditional local brew of beetroot wine, and recipes are guarded jealously.

Beet went into folk use as a medicine, but was rarely used as a vegetable. Gerard wrote:

What might be made of the red and beautifull roote, I refer unto the curious and cunning Cooke, who no doubt when he hath had the view thereof, and is assured that it is both good and holsome, will make thereof many and divers dishes both faire and good.

The famous royal gardener, Tradescant the Younger, imported improved varieties of beet from Germany in about 1656. After King Charles I was beheaded, Oliver Cromwell came to power as Lord Protector of England and ordered that the palace gardens be turned over to 'serious pursuits and the growing of vegetables'.

Cromwell thoroughly approved of the earthy red beets, and soon no frugal Puritan feast in England was complete without side dishes of beets sliced in vinegar. The rich sugar content had been isolated in Germany in the mid-eighteenth century, but little notice was taken of this until France and Britain were in the grip of the savage years of the Napoleonic Wars. France was feeling the effects of the British naval blockade, so French chemists started extracting the sugar from beet on a large scale. Napoleon encouraged this wholeheartedly, in fact, he gave priority to the project. Perhaps he wanted to keep the people sweet!

> **Folk Use** <

In France, red beet juice has been valued as a fine liver detoxificant since medieval times. One week a year is traditionally set aside to rest the liver. During this time, a wineglassful of raw beet juice is drunk each morning on an empty stomach. Throughout the day, beet juice is taken instead of alcohol in moderate amounts of about 200 ml. Palatable beet juice is made by baking the beets, peeling and chopping them into small pieces. Put these through either a sieve or a blender and mix with water or mineral water.

In Germany and Poland beet roots and juices are used almost daily to build up the body's resistance. The Poles also use beet as medicine *after* a serious illness, to cleanse the toxins out of the system. A fermented beet dish, quite similar to the Russian *kvas*, is fed to people fatigued or run-down after an illness.

In the North East of England a traditional pick-me-up is drunk throughout the first week of spring to 'get winter out of the body'. It consists of equal amounts of celery juice, beet juice, carrot juice and sarsaparilla.

Beet has always been used in folk medicine to keep the blood in good condition. Beet juices and teas are traditionally given to anyone suffering from anaemia. Again this shows the infinite wisdom and observation of the folk plant heritage, especially since we now know beet leaves to be one of the richest sources of iron.

Beet juices are also taken to fight acidity, and as a dietary aid for low blood pressure.

Beet leaf tea is a fine remedy for female troubles. Women in Poland, Russia and Germany, especially those of child-bearing age, take regular monthly courses of the tea to keep the reproductive system in good order. Folk users believe that beet leaf tea helps fertility and prevents problem periods.

Beet leaf tea is also taken for jaundice and to relieve liver congestion, or any problems in that area. It is made in this way: chop two cups of clean beet leaves finely and put them in a saucepan. Pour over eight cups of cold water and bring to the boil. Hold the heat for one minute, then allow to stand, covered, for 10 minutes. Drink six cups of beet leaf tea a day, either warm or cold, for a total of six days.

> Herbal Medicine <

The early English herbalists had a high regard for beet juice. Culpeper said that it was 'good for the headache and swimmings therein and all affectations of the brain'. He also said: 'It is good for all weals, pushes, blisters and blains in the skin: the decoction in water and vinegar healeth the itch if bathed therewith and cleanseth the head of dandriff, scurf and dry scabs and relieves running sores and ulcers and is much commended against baldness and shedding the hair.' Gerard found that the juice expressed from the roots and leaves was 'of a cleansing, digestive quality'. The old herbalists also recommended beet juice to 'stay the bloody flux' and to 'help the yellow jaundice'.

Strangely enough, beets have since lost their place in English herbal medicine. European registered medical herbalists, however, still retain a very high opinion of the therapeutic powers of beet juices and teas. They treat cirrhosis of the liver with beet leaf tea and courses of beet juices. Beet juice is also used to counteract the effects of over-rich food and drinks. It is a standard remedy for liverish chills and biliousness.

>• Homeopathic Medicine <

Homeopathic doctors in Germany prescribe red beet juice for many cases of jaundice, hepatitis and other serious liver complaints. They also recommend it to correct faulty fat absorption and biliary insufficiency. Dr F. Keital of Berlin has perfected a lactic fermentation of beet juice which preserves all the remarkable active medicinal principles. This beet juice tastes quite delicious and is now widely available in specialist stores around the world.

> Culinary Use <

Baking beet roots rather than boiling them preserves more of the active constituents. Of course, a dish like the superb Ukrainian beet *kvas* has its own medicinal values. *Kvas* is made from fermented beets and is popularly used in *borsch*, to which it imparts a pleasant mellow flavour. *Kvas* is made by putting chopped beets into an earthenware crock and covering them with boiled water which has been cooled to lukewarm. Slices of sour rye bread are pressed over the beets and the container is covered and kept at room temperature for a few days. The fermented liquid is drunk as a beverage or poured into *borsch*.

Traditional Ukrainian *borsch* is made with beets, carrots, potatoes and cabbage, all finely shredded, mixed with cooked white beans, chopped dill, beet *kvas* or lemon juice, and sour cream.

In the summer, a fine chilled beet root soup can be made with shredded beets, chicken stock, the juice of one orange and a carton of yogurt.

In Scandinavia, shredded beet is mixed with minced meat to make meatballs. The Finns use cooked beet root with their fish salads, adding gherkins and vinaigrette dressing.

From the U.S.A. we have many imaginative beet recipes, including cooked beet root with orange, beet with apple, beet savoury toast with roll mop herrings and hard-boiled eggs, spiced beet with cinnamon, and beet root in yogurt with chives, cinnamon and nutmeg.

To get a really good flavour, try wrapping well scrubbed beet root in foil and baking it in a moderate oven for about two hours, depending on the size. A quick cooking method, and one that retains nutritional values, is to shred raw beet root into a saucepan, add a minute amount of water and one tablespoon of olive or sunflower oil. Clamp on a tight-fitting lid and simmer on a low heat for about 20 minutes. This can be served with nutmeg and sour cream. Grated raw beet root can also be brushed with oil and baked in the oven for about 20 minutes. Alternatively it can be baked in milk.

Beet leaves can be used very much like spinach, that is, braised or steamed. It is best to cut out the thick lower rib, as this tends to be tough.

Raw beet has a distinctive earthy taste but don't be put off. Raw beet can taste delicious grated very finely, dressed with a cream sauce or mayonnaise and flavoured with lovage, thyme and caraway seeds.

> BEVERAGES <

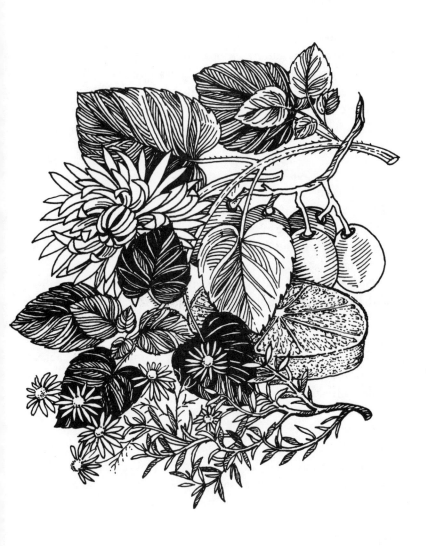

> Fruit Juices <

Fresh juices are an excellent source of vitamins, minerals and enzymes, and are so quickly absorbed by the body that they are an ideal way of treating yourself to the health-giving qualities of the plant. It is far better to drink fresh, raw juice because active enzymes are destroyed at temperatures over 140°F. (60°C.) which means, of course, that commercially canned and bottled juices have lost their enzymes.

Many people find an electric juicer a good investment for health. It delivers full nutritional value of the fruit or vegetable with the exception of fibre which it neatly extracts. The fibrous part left over after juicing need not be wasted. It makes a tasty dessert or soup base.

Two fruit juices deserve special mention here for their unusual benefits:

> Grape juice <

The grape cure is perhaps the most popular of all natural diet therapies. The vine was one of the first fruits to be grown by primitive man, and its long, impressive folk use as a medicine has been substantiated by clinical observation this century.

Grape diets and fasts are immensely popular at European spas and have been thoroughly applied at the Bircher-Benner clinic at Zurich for over fifty years. Health farms around the world use the grape cure with noticeable effect.

Grape's secret lies somewhere in its combination of natural constituents. It contains dextrose and fructose, mineral salts, malic and tartaric acid, tannin, pectin, phosphorus, flavone glycosides, pigment and the vitamins A, B, and C.

Grape has long been observed for its tonic effect, and it also acts on the bowels and kidneys which are stimulated to eliminate waste and toxins. Under medical supervision, grape juices and fasts are used to treat liver disorders, constipation and obesity.

At spas or health farms it is obviously possible to keep on the grape diet under supervision for a week or more, but that is not advisable at home. Happily, the grape cure does adapt easily and safely to home use because one or two days are enough for the special actions to start working.

In fact, Dr Bircher-Benner advised a 'grape day', during which about two pounds of grapes were divided into four or five portions and eaten instead of meals. This is recommended as safe enough for pregnant women and overweight people with other health problems.

Other doctors allow their grape cure dieters and patients to eat up to four pounds of grapes a day, or two pounds of grapes and one litre of grape juice (which must be free from additional sugar and additives).

Grapes are so rich in dextrose and fructose that it might be surprising to learn that they are a respected slimming aid. The answer lies in the richness of natural sugars which keep the dieter from feeling those terrible pangs of hunger which wrack so many other day-long fasts.

Where grapes are used as a medicinal cure they must be very carefully washed to remove sprays. Soak a pound of grapes in the juice of half a lemon for four or five minutes then rinse again before eating.

> Lemon juice <

Lemon juice is a powerful and agreeable natural antiseptic. In French experiments last century, lemon juice was shown to neutralize various bacteria, including typhoid, in periods ranging from 20 to 180 minutes.

We have always instinctively valued the anti-bacterial power of lemon. In fact, our custom of eating a slice of lemon with fish is a preventative measure rather than decorative. Similarly, we are using lemon juice's antiseptic protection when we sprinkle it on oysters or other shellfish.

Lemon's rich content of vitamin C saved countless sailors

from the curse of scurvy over several centuries. Its germicidal action and the vitamin C content make lemon juice an ideal remedy during colds or flu. The time-honoured treatment is to retire to bed and sip the juice of a lemon mixed with a little water and a dessertspoon of honey, with perhaps a nip of brandy. Diluted, cold (not iced) lemon juice is very thirst-quenching and cooling when the sufferer is feverish. It was used to reduce the raging temperatures of malaria when quinine was in short supply.

For sore throats, dilute the juice of a lemon with the same amount of water and gargle every two hours.

Lemon juice has traditionally been taken to treat rheumatism, stubborn hiccoughs, jaundice and stomach ache.

A recent successful advertising campaign has persuaded would-be dieters that lemon juice is slimming. In fact, strong lemon juice is very stimulating to the whole system, so slimmers should beware of exciting their gastric juices!

Lemon juice has been a popular beauty aid for centuries. It is used, slightly salted, as a lotion to make freckles disappear, or mixed with glycerine to soften and whiten hands. Lemon juice is excellent for bringing back the highlights to faded blonde hair or for brightening honest 'mouse'. Put undiluted lemon juice on your hair and sit in the sun, then shampoo.

> **Herb Teas** <

The most familiar method of making herb tea is by *infusion*. It is very simple. A teaspoon of dried herbs is placed in a previously warmed cup or teapot and boiling water is added. The infusion is covered and left to stand for about five minutes, then strained, and lemon or honey is added to taste.

A *decoction* is made of plant materials – such as seeds, twigs or roots – which are not so easy to extract. A teaspoon of the dried material is placed in an enamel saucepan (never a metal one) with about one cup of water, brought to the boil and then simmered for three minutes. The liquid is strained and sweetened. Decoctions are much more powerful than infusions and should only be taken for short periods.

A *maceration* is used when the herbs contain a high proportion of volatile oils and mucilage. A teaspoon of dried herbs is placed in a cupful of cold water or alcohol and left to steep for at least twelve hours at room temperature. The resulting mixture is then warmed, strained, and sweetened to taste.

Herb teas are now widely available in quick and easy teabag form. The old favourites chamomile, lime and mint are a good introduction for the faint-hearted who have never tried herb teas. Another way to acquire the taste is to add a teaspoon of dried herbs to the ordinary India or China blend of tea leaves.

When herb teas are taken specifically as a medicine they are taken two or three times a day, after meals, for a period of one to two months. Listed below are the most frequently prescribed herb teas, all of which are suitable for home use. Seeds such as celery or caraway should be well bruised or crushed before being added to boiling water.

Suggested herb tea	Complaint
Alfalfa leaves and seeds	Lack of vitality
Angelica root	Headaches Exhaustion
Anise seeds	Gastric and intestinal disorders
Balm leaves	Sleeplessness Headache
Basil	Fatigue General debility
Buchu leaves	Cystitis Bladder problems
Caraway seeds	Flatulence
Celery seed and leaves	Arthritis Rheumatism

Eat Your Way to Health

Chamomile blossoms	Eczema
	Jittery nerves
	Sleeplessness
	Colds
	Menstrual pain
Dandelion root and leaves	Kidney and liver problems
	Constipation
Dill seeds	Flatulence
	Restless babies
Elder blossoms and leaves	Chills
	Fevers
	Colds
Fennel seeds and leaves	Eye problems
	Indigestion
	Coughs
Fenugreek seed	Underweight
	General debility
Ginseng	Lack of vitality
Hawthorn blossoms	Nervous stress
Hops	Sleeplessness
	Nervous tension
	Irritability
Iceland Moss	Diarrhoea
	Chronic catarrh
Lady's Mantle	Menstrual disorders
Lavender	Fainting
	Headache
Licorice root	Gastric ulcers
	Bronchitis
Lime blossoms	Chills
	Influenza
Marjoram leaves	Digestive complaints
	Aching joints

Mint leaves	Flatulence
	Gastritis
	Nausea
Mullein blossoms	Coughs
	Bronchitis
Nettle leaves	Bladder troubles
	Rheumatism
	Arthritis
Raspberry leaves	Menstrual disorders
	Morning sickness
Sage leaves	Sore throats
	Coughs
	Hair loss
Sarsaparilla root	Lack of virility
Senna pods	Chronic constipation
Thyme	Colds
	Respiratory infections
	Indigestion
Sweet cicely	Exhaustion
	Problems of puberty

> Other Health Drinks <

> Alternative teas <

Bancha tea is a macrobiotic tea made from herbs and twigs. George Ohsawa, who introduced macrobiotics to the U.S.A., recommends ten parts of bancha tea to one part of soy sauce for an instant 'pick-me-up'.

Green buckwheat tea is made from natural dried buckwheat blossom and leaf and contains all the benefits of the plant. Buckwheat is rich in rutin which has an excellent effect on the arteries and circulation. It is also rich in iron and B vitamins. Buckwheat tea is free from caffeine and tannin which can cause digestive imbalances.

Gossip tea is made from rosehips, cloves, orange peel, and hibiscus and has a spicy flavour. It is rich in vitamin C and tannin-free.

Luaka tea comes from the high mountainous regions in the east of Sri Lanka. It is lower in tannin and caffeine than other usual tea blends.

Mu tea is the great Japanese tea which contains ginseng and fifteen other herbs, including licorice root, coptis, rehmannia, paonia root, and hoelen. The word 'mu' is Japanese for infinity or space. Macrobiotic enthusiasts think highly of this tea. It has a rounded, spicy taste and is a powerful stimulant.

Rooibosch tea comes from the *Aspalathus limearis* plant, which grows on the sloping mountains of the West Cape in South Africa. It contains no caffeine or tannin, and many claims are made for its health-giving properties, especially for those who are allergic to ordinary teas. Rooibosch tea contains vitamin C, iron, manganese, calcium, magnesium, potassium and sulphur. The Hottentot tribes first discovered the healing powers of this tea. It has a pleasant taste, not unlike Earl Grey, and is distributed world-wide.

> > Coffee substitutes <

Dandelion coffee is one of the most delicious of the coffee substitutes. It can be bought commercially as an instant powder, but is very easy to make yourself. Dig up the roots of two-year-old dandelion plants in autumn when they are stocked with essential food reserves. Snip off the leaves, wash the roots gently and pat dry with kitchen paper. Bake them in a moderate oven for several hours until the familiar roast smell fills the kitchen. Chop the roast roots and grind them in a coffee grinder; for a really flavoursome coffee, put these granules in a hot oven again for a few minutes to toast them to fine flavour. The roasted and ground roots will keep well in airtight jars.

Grain coffees include many ingenious mixtures based on toasted grains. One popular variety contains rye, oats, millet, barley, figs and chicory. Another, widely used, is made from toasted bran, wheat and molasses. These grain beverages are natural laxatives and need gentle boiling to bring out the flavour. They actually improve with reheating.

Postum is the original coffee substitute and deserves a special mention. It is difficult to make at home. The manufacturers make it by mixing molasses and bran and roasting them to a high temperature. Red wheat is then blended in, and the ingredients finely ground. Boiling water is added to this mixture to make a tasty drink with diuretic properties.

> ❯ High protein drinks ❮

These drinks are made by mixing natural food protein powders with milk or water. The powders contain a wide variety of ingredients: typical constituents are lecithin granules, brewers yeast, vegetable oils such as safflower and sunflower, carob, dried yogurt, papaya enzyme, with vitamin and mineral powders. It is often cheaper to buy the ingredients and mix the drinks yourself.

The value of high protein drinks lies in their concentration and balance of essential nutrients. During illness or times of stress, each item of the drink can be carefully chosen for its specific properties. These concentrated drinks can take the place of a meal when time is short, for example, at breakfast.

> ❯ Lemon and barley water ❮

The famous Miss Crawford, governess to Her Majesty the Queen, has been quoted as saying that the Royal Family owe their superb complexions to their habit of drinking lemon and barley water daily. Barley water is mildly diuretic and excellent for any urinary troubles. It is a very soothing drink and a definite aid to the digestion, and is traditionally given to babies who cannot tolerate milk. Lemon and barley water is a fine drink to take during influenza or colds because it acts on catarrh and helps the body cope with fevers.

One old-fashioned and good-tasting recipe uses 50 grams of pearl barley to half a litre of water. Wash the barley well, then add the water and bring quickly to the boil. Simmer slowly for half an hour, strain, and add the juice of one lemon and honey to taste. The barley need not be thrown away. It can be used like rice.

>   Mineral waters   <

Bottled waters from recognized springs and sources are the most beneficial of all waters. As the name suggests, they are rich sources of minerals. Many natural springs provide calcium, iron, magnesium, manganese, zinc and other trace minerals. Several countries have outstandingly good springs which are strictly controlled by government authorities. France has the great three, Vichy, Volvic and Perrier. Many medicinal claims have been made for these waters, and it is possible that they aid digestion and stomach troubles as well as providing essential trace minerals. Volvic is said to be so pure that it can be given to babies without sterilization. Certainly French maternity hospitals are very keen on training mothers to give their babies mineral waters rather than tap water as they grow up.

Queen Elizabeth II drinks only Malvern water, which is bottled at the pure spring at Malvern in the West of England. Crates of this mineral water accompany her on trips abroad.

Each bottle of mineral water should state quite clearly any mineral content and whether it has been approved by a government body. Experiment with the various mineral waters cheaply available and find the one which suits you best.

❯ Rosehip syrup ❮

Rosehips are very high in vitamin C and the syrup has demulcent or soothing properties. All in all, a delightful and cheap home remedy to make yourself.

Gather the hips before they grow too soft and take off the heads and stalks. Slit the hips in half and remove all the seeds and whites. Press them through a sieve or put them in the blender. Add their own weight in sugar and enough water to make a syrup. Bring slowly to the boil and simmer, stirring all the time, until the mixture is really soft and syrupy. Strain if necessary, then store in clean bottles with well-fitting lids.

❯ Rice water ❮

Rice water has a very calming effect on the digestive tract and is also useful for urinary troubles. At a London maternity hospital in 1965, many newborn babies became sick during an outbreak of gastritis. One of the hospital paediatricians had seen rice water used as a medicinal treatment in India. He prescribed minute amounts of it for the babies and the sickness soon stopped.

To make rice water, use two tablespoons of rice (preferably brown organically grown rice) to one litre of water. Bring quickly to a rolling boil, then put a lid on and simmer for about 30 minutes. Strain and cool before use.

❮ Ginger beer ❯

Ginger beer is the homemade alcoholic beverage highly prized by the Chinese for its cold- and flu-preventing properties. Take 450 grams of brown sugar, 25 grams of bruised ginger root, and a pinch of hops and saffron (optional). Add five litres of water and boil for a few minutes. Then add another eight litres of water and a tablespoon of fresh yeast or wine yeast. Let the mixture work all night and bear in mind that it will effervesce or fizz almost like champagne. Next morning pour into sterilized bottles, leaving plenty of room for expansion. Do not cork for several days.

> Wine <

It would be so pleasant to think that the wine we drink for pleasure was actually doing us a power of good at the same time. Indeed, the respected French homeopathic doctor, E. A. Maury, has written a book enticingly called *Wine is the Best Medicine* (published by Corgi Books, 1978).

Dr Maury points out in his book that wine contains rich quantities of trace minerals, including iron and calcium, and that it is a natural antiseptic.

He believes that the right wine, carefully chosen, can treat a variety of ailments such as arthritis, cystitis, diarrhoea, nervous depression, eczema, and many others.

Naturally, Dr Maury thinks we should treat the wine with respect and drink moderate amounts of the wines he details.

One problem most of us have is to buy wine which has not been chemically treated. One good way round this is to make your own wine at home. Traditionally, home-made wines have been greatly valued as medicines. Alcohol provides a superb base for preserving the medicinal qualities of the fruit or vegetable. Many of the items of which I have given detailed descriptions in this book can be made into excellent wine: beetroot, potato, honey, black currant, blackberry or celery. Others such as elderberry, ginger or rhubarb have their own individual properties.

Country folk have always used their kitchen wines (often highly potent) as an aid to health and a preventative medicine.

Good medicated wine can be quickly made in this way: to two litres of good red wine, add a sprig of rosemary, a sprig of wormwood, six cherries, two whole nutmegs, an inch of cinnamon bark, a small piece of bruised root ginger and about ten large raisins. Put the wine in a warm place for about a week and shake it every day. Strain, add some more plain red wine to the mixture and drink it after meals as a tonic.

> BLACK CURRANT <

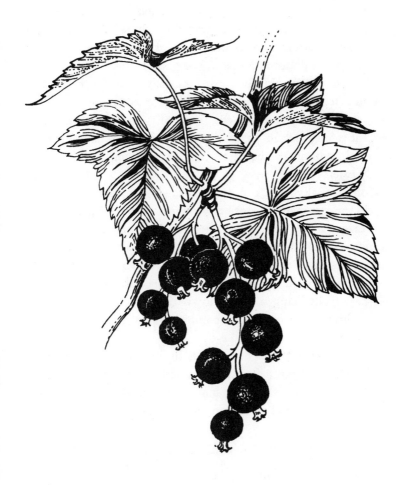

> Health <

Anyone who has ever sucked a black currant pastille or lozenge knows its soothing effect on sore throats and irritating coughs. Black currant is very popular with doctors in France, who advise a tisane (tea) made of the leaves to soothe acidity, break up a cold, and quench thirst during fever. Black currant leaves also have a diuretic effect. In the dark days of rationing in Britain in the 1940s, old age pensioners gathered black currant leaves to supplement their allowance of 'India blend' tea. This was a good tasting combination and, of course, made a cheap tea, which no doubt did a power of good to their kidneys.

Modern pharmacists use black currant fruit for two main reasons: to flavour medicines, syrups, lozenges and pastilles; and as a dietary supplement, especially for children. Black currant is very rich in vitamin C and its delicious flavour makes an ideal addition to the diet of babies, growing children, and faddy eaters.

Commercially, black currant cordials are sold around the world under many proprietary brand names. Each national pharmacopoeia lays down quality standards. In most countries permitted food dyes may be added to the black currant pulp before it is made into cordial or juices. Natural juices or syrups without any colouring can be found in specialist food stores.

Apart from being a well-known rich source of vitamin C, black currant also contains a combination of fruit acids, pectin and rutin.

The red currant (*Ribes rubrum*) is similar in medicinal virtues to the black currant, except that it does not possess the same curative powers for the throat and mouth. However, red currant (which can be white) is more powerfully laxative.

> Constituents <

The ascorbic acid content of the ripe fruit varies from 100 to 300 mg in each 100 grams. It also contains citric and malic acid, pectin, rutin, potassium, calcium, iron and sulphur. The leaves contain organic acids, tannin, volatile oil, and enzyme emulsion.

> History <

The black currant which is now cultivated commercially all around the world is native to Britain and Northern Europe. It grows naturally in damp woods.

The black fruit was not so popular with the early English herbalists as the red currant and white currant. Gerard described the black fruit as 'of a stinking and somewhat loathing savour'. Black currant does have a distinctive woody smell. In spite of this, it has always been popular as a folk medicine and a fruit, and it was one of those taken by early settlers to America and Australia.

> Folk Use <

Black currant juice has been a favourite remedy for quinsy and sore throats for five centuries. Folk use here closely parallels modern herbal practice, since black currant is used as a popular remedy for sore throats, hoarseness, and colds with temperatures. Until the First World War, great use was made of black currant jellies for soothing sore throats, and as a food during fevers. Children who breathed through their mouths instead of their noses were traditionally made to eat black currant jelly.

The fresh juice is deservedly popular for its thirst-quenching qualities, especially nice for parched throats. Folk medicine used the rich vitamin C content to treat scurvy, pregnancy disorders, and some cases of anaemia. It proved to be so valuable in reducing high fevers that it was known for centuries as 'quinsy berry'.

Black currant leaf tea is traditionally used to prevent prostate gland troubles, which is why it is generally considered a male medicine in Britain. French folk use has no such discrimination and has made the most of the diuretic properties of the leaves, which are made into tisanes for many urinary disorders such as cystitis and retention of urine.

> Herbal Medicine <

Fresh black currant juice is valued by herbalists for its beneficial action on the throat and mouth. It is particularly recommended when sore throats and colds are accompanied by high temperatures or fever. Black currant juice is noted to have a soothing effect on sore or inflamed throats. It is an excellent anti-fever agent, especially drunk hot, when it promotes sweating. All in all it is a valuable aid against feverish colds.

An infusion of black currant leaves is used herbally as a diuretic and especially prescribed when cleansing action is needed, such as when toxins remain in the body following serious illness.

In herbal medicine, the ripe currants are known as refrigerant – a delightful and very modern word which describes the cooling properties. Sore throats with a slight rise in temperature can be treated with a wine glass of fresh juice taken every hour for four hours. A hot syrup or cordial is most beneficial at bedtime, and may be made quickly and easily by pouring boiling water onto good black currant jam. Add the juice of half a lemon and honey to flavour.

> Culinary Use <

Delicious jams, purées, cordials, juices, syrups, wines and liqueurs are made with black currant. In France a popular liqueur (*liqueur de cassis*) is made with one kilo of black currants, one teaspoon (2 grams) each of cloves and cinnamon, three litres of spirits, 750 grams of sugar, and a few black currant leaves if available. Put the ingredients into a crockery or stone jar, mix every day for a fortnight, then strain, filter, and bottle. The French also make a delicious black currant wine in much the same way, using much less sugar.

For black currant tea, gather the leaves after flowering and before the berries ripen. Dry in the shade, or a cool place in the kitchen. Use half to one teaspoon of leaves to each cup of boiling water, and stand or infuse for about three minutes. A very simple way to put black currant leaves into everyday use is to add them, like the old age pensioners did in Britain during rationing, to Indian, Chinese or herbal teas.

> BLACKBERRY <

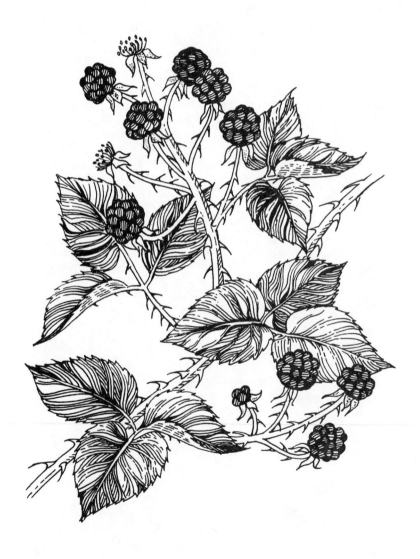

> Health <

The thorny blackberry bramble which obligingly grows wild in any climate is a valuable 'food for free'. Every part of the bush has medicinal value: the root is astringent, the leaves contain tannin and are tonic and astringent, the fruits (the familiar berries) are tonic and rich in vitamin C. Green berries, ripe blackberries and even blossom appear on the bramble at the same time – an unusual sight in nature. The ripe berry is laxative, but the green berry has the opposite effect and can be used to combat diarrhoea. This explains the seemingly conflicting advice in the old herbals which could assume such knowledge on the part of readers.

Over-ripe berries can be indigestible, a point on which the old herbalists were quite explicit. It was, in fact, an old English belief that the Devil defiled all blackberries at Michaelmas by spitting on them. Autumn blackberry pickers will know the oozing, slightly fermenting look of over-ripe berries.

Bramble bushes' tonic and astringent qualities have been appreciated for centuries, but modern research in the last decade has added another dimension. Blackberries are surprisingly high in natural fibre, which we all now know to be essential for good health.

Opinions still differ as to whether there is one true blackberry or many varieties. The same botanical family furnishes dewberry (*Rubus coesius*), cloudberry (*R. chamoenorus*), and the American bramble (*R. odoratus*). The American blackberry (*R. villosus*) is a first cousin. All the family share the medicinal properties and have similar actions.

> Constituents <

The fruit or berry contains malic and citric acid, pectin, vitamin C, iron, potassium, calcium, sulphur and magnesium. It is an excellent source of fibre, about four grams in each 100 grams (or about three-quarters of an average breakfast cup).

The leaves contain tannin, and a natural astringent. The bark and roots contain tannin and a strong astringent principle.

> History <

Blackberry bramble bushes have become entwined in popular mythology as a protection or charm against 'evil runes'. In the highlands of Scotland blackberry is *an druise beannaichte*, the blessed bramble.

It was with a bramble that Christ drove the moneylenders out of the temple and later switched the donkey to Jerusalem. This scriptural pedigree has, no doubt, been responsible for the magical or blessed image of the bramble bush and may have prompted some of the folk uses.

> Folk Use <

The American Shakers of the last century made particularly interesting medicinal use of this fruit. Surprisingly, this sincere religious group made the fruit into delicious, heady wines and brandies as well as the usual cordials and infusions.

Shaker blackberry remedies were used to treat dysentery, infant cholera, prolapsed conditions, and bad breath. In this the Shakers showed their understanding of the tonic and astringent properties of blackberry.

Traditional English uses of blackberry brambles were often weird and wonderful or merely furtive. Creeping under a bramble bush was a popular charm against rheumatism and boils. Children with hernias were passed ritually under a branching bramble. Unfortunate cows with the staggers were dragged under bramble loops. In spite of these customs, intelligent folk remedies still exist today. Fresh blackberry juice or wine is used as a nerve tonic, a laxative, or a gargle for sore throats and gums. In France, a tisane of blackberry blossoms is used as a douche for female problems such as the whites (leucorrhoea).

In bygone years, a popular European hair dye was made by boiling blackberry leaves in strong lye (the alkaline extract of wood ash in water) to make a permanent, soft dark hair colour. An infusion of the leaves alone will colour the hair. The roots were boiled to make an orange dye for clothes.

> **Herbal Medicine** <

Ripe blackberry is recognized as strongly eliminative and used to flush toxins from the system. The raw berries are recommended for their laxative powers and their general tonic effect.

The leaves are valued for their astringent properties and prescribed for leucorrhoea and profuse menses. Blackberry leaves are considered to be one of the best remedies for diarrhoea in childhood.

An infusion, or simple blackberry leaf tea is made in much the usual way, with about one teaspoon of fresh or dried leaves to one cup of boiling water. The dose varies according to age – one teaspoon four or five times a day will often be sufficient for young children, while adults might need one cup three times a day.

This blackberry tea is considered very beneficial to the mucous membranes and intestinal muscles. It is also taken hot for colds, and warm as a gargle for sore throats.

> **Culinary Use** <

Blackberry is familiar in jams and jellies but it is also delicious in cordials, syrups and wines. A nutritious syrup is made by cooking the slightly under-ripe blackberries in equal weights of their own juice. Honey or sugar is added to taste.

In France a delicious liqueur is made by steeping one large handful of ripe blackberries in one litre of alcohol (white wine would do well). The mixture is left on a window sill in the sun or near a hot stove for three weeks, and stirred occasionally. It is then filtered, and sweetened, to become a delicious and medicinal liqueur.

For the best benefits from blackberry tea, gather the young shoots in spring, soon after the leaves unfurl. Dry them as you would any herb, and brew up into a pleasant tea with many medicinal qualities.

❯ BRAN ❮

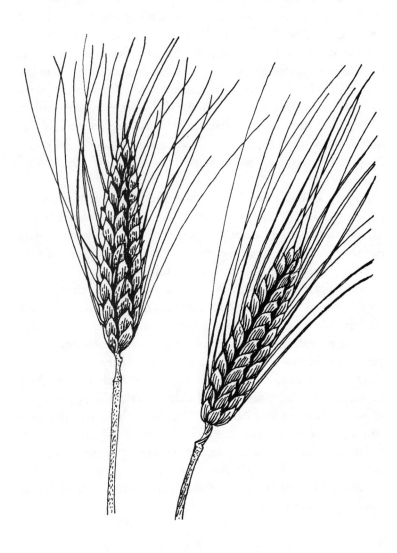

Bran is the one healthy food that we all know about. You would have to be an Aboriginal nomad wandering in the vast Australian deserts to have escaped the media message that bran is *good*. Our doctors talk about stool transit times with the happy air of airport officials announcing departures. Leading specialists tell us that a dessertspoon of bran can transform our lives and prevent many of the ills that Western civilization is prey to.

What most people do not realize is that this evangelical zeal represents a complete volte-face by orthodox medicine. Late last century, in the 1880s, Dr T. R. Allinson warned that the removal of bran and wheat germ from the daily bread would lead to widespread degenerative diseases. His colleagues greeted his statements with derision, but Dr Allinson refused to be silent. Finally, he was labelled a crank and struck off the medical register.

As late as the 1960s one leading specialist was treating his patients on a high fibre diet in strict secret for fear of ridicule by his colleagues. Not so long ago, health food enthusiasts who openly piled their cereal bowls with bran were asked incredulously: 'Are you going to *eat* that stuff?'

Gradually, not dramatically, the climate began to change. The food pioneer Sir Robert McCarrison did his famous research into the Hunza and Sikh diets in the 1930s. Sir Robert's opinions were respected, and when he advocated wholemeal flour complete with bran a few enlightened people listened.

Then, in America during the 1950s, the Kellogg Company sponsored detailed studies at Michigan State College into the effects of their product All-Bran. This research showed that bran had a profound laxative effect and that fibre (which used to be called 'roughage') was essential in preventing constipation. The Michigan researchers felt that bran might also prevent certain 'civilized' diseases such as appendicitis and diverticulitis and they urged further trials.

A whole series of tests followed in the U.S.A. At the U.S. Department of Agriculture laboratory in North Dakota it was found that cereal bran significantly lowered cholesterol levels. Many other researchers in the U.S.A. have since proved that blood cholesterol levels fall when people eat fibre-rich foods.

At Washington, a study showed that fibre also offers another valuable protection. Fibre has the ability to absorb chemicals such as cyclamates, additives, and other toxic substances and expel them from the body. This has the tremendous potential of rendering the bowel less susceptible to disease.

U.S. researchers have also done fascinating research into immigrants, sometimes 'pairing' them with brothers or sisters back home still eating traditional diets. In several surveys, Japanese, Irish and Italian immigrants who had adopted a typical refined American diet were shown to suffer much more heart disease than their relatives eating fibre-rich diets in the home country.

In Britain, Denis P. Burkitt, M.D., F.R.C.S., Senior Research Fellow in Geographical Pathology at St Thomas's Hospital, London, is the leading spokesman on bran and health. When Dr Burkitt addressed a conference in London, health food stores all over the country sold out of bran overnight.

Dr Burkitt believes that a formidable list of so-called civilized diseases can be prevented by the regular use of bran. These include: diverticulitis (a balloon-type blow-out of the colon wall), appendicitis, hiatus hernia, varicose veins, haemorrhoids, cancer of the large intestine and bowel, heart disease and gall-stones.

Transit time — or the length of time it takes the food residue to pass through the gut — is believed to be a vital clue to low-fibre related illnesses. In affluent Western countries, transit time is usually twice as long as in rural Africa or India.

To the Zulus a long transit time is two days; an average medium-fibre Western diet transit takes five days; in old people on very refined diets, transit has been known to take two weeks.

The dangers of this are obvious. Dr Burkitt says: 'On a high-fibre diet poisonous substances will be diluted and washed out every day. We believe that bowel cancer is caused by carcinogenous substances in the faeces acting in the gut.'

If, then, fibre is an essential part of the healthy diet, what exactly is it and how should we eat it every day?

Dietary fibre is the group of complex substances found in plant cells which the human digestive enzymes cannot break down. Cereal fibre is different to fruit and vegetable fibre, but the latest thinking is that our bodies are actually programmed to deal with a combination of these fibres. So an ideal diet would contain a balanced variety of cereal, such as bran fibre, and fruit and vegetable fibres. It is as well to remember that eggs, fish, meat, milk, sugar, fats and alcoholic drinks contain no dietary fibre whatsoever.

Dr Burkitt advises us to take one dessertspoon of bran a day for good functioning. More than that is not needed and should not be used except when the bran is being taken medically to treat diverticulitis or other problems. Bran absorbs water in the colon, so people who put dry bran powder or flakes on top of their cereal should be sure to take extra liquid as well.

To get the balance of the different fibres make daily use of fibre-rich fruit and vegetables such as onions, cabbages, potatoes, carrots, turnips, apples, bananas, avocados, fresh blackberries, papaya, dates, figs, strawberries and raspberries.

Quite the simplest way to put cereal fibre into your daily life is to eat only wholemeal bread, but beware, not all bread sold as brown contains bran. If you buy 100 percent wholemeal bread, you are sure of getting a bran content.

Often someone will say: 'But bran and wholemeal bread just do not agree with me.' Start slowly with small amounts. It often takes the system two or three weeks to adjust to a higher fibre intake. Until the adjustment is made you may feel unpleasantly flatulent or gassy and have mild diarrhoea.

> Bran and Slimming <

Many people are reluctant to adopt bran wholeheartedly because they fear it will make them put on weight. You can actually lose weight on a high-fibre diet provided you follow these simple rules:

Cut out or drastically reduce sugar in your diet.

Cut out all refined carbohydrates (white flour, white rice, white sugar and anything made with them such as biscuits or cakes).

Reduce your daily intake of fat and salt.

Don't take pop or fizzy drinks.

Eat more raw fruit and vegetables.

High-fibre diets are so filling and satisfying that you will not find it hard to cut these things out of daily use. The weight loss will be gradual and the health benefits enormous.

> Constituents <

One dessertspoon (approximately one gram) of bran flakes or bran powder provides .05 grams of fibre. It also contains iron, calcium, potassium, and traces of B vitamins.

> History <

The first wheat began to grow at least 10,000 years ago in the fertile crescent surrounding the eastern Mediterranean. Man's skills in grinding and storing the grain eventually led to a more settled way of life. By about 4000 B.C. the early Egyptians had brought wheat cooking to a fine art. They isolated yeast as the mysterious ingredient which could cause the dough to rise. In their clay ovens, the Egyptians baked exotic high-rising domed, coiled and plaited bread, and Egypt became the grain basket for the Roman Empire. The majority of Cleopatra's 'treacherous vessels' were used for carrying wheat to Rome. In turn the wheat seeds were taken to Britain and Gaul by the Roman legions.

Over a thousand years later, in 1493, Columbus carried wheat grains with him to the West Indies; Cortes took wheat with him to Mexico in 1519. During the whole period of English colonialization wheat grains were shipped to Australia, North America, and South Africa.

It is a tribute to this truly versatile grass plant that it has grown and flourished in every climate.

> Folk Use <

Our ancestors were well aware of the laxative qualities of bran. A fourteenth-century recipe, describing how to make brown bread for servants, starts with these words:

Browne breade made of the coarsest of wheat having in it much branne, filleth the belly with excrements ... and besides that, it is good for labourers, I have known that such as have been used to fine bread, when they have been costive [constipated], by eating browne bread and butter have been made soluble.

Bran was also employed for an extraordinary variety of purposes. It was used for washing seventeenth-century chintz, stuffing upholstery, dry-shampooing hair and feeding animals.

It is still highly valued as a beauty treatment and used with water as a soap substitute or complexion scrub, or mixed with buttermilk or lemon juice to treat oily skins and enlarged pores. Bran flakes or powder are also used as an all-over cleanser and softener. Throw a handful in the bath when the water is running and rub a dampened handful all over your body.

Traditionally, bran tea is given to weakly children and adults, and in cases of anaemia, continual colds, catarrh, weak digestion, sluggish kidneys, bronchitis and general run-down feelings.

Bran tea is made by adding two heaped tablespoons of clean bran flakes to three quarters of a litre of boiling water. Simmer for 15 minutes, strain and flavour with lemon or honey.

> **Herbal Medicine** <

Bran provides an excellent illustration of the importance that sound nutrition plays in alternative medicine. Many herbalists and naturopaths question a patient closely about his diet and advise an adjustment of the daily fibre intake before beginning a course of treatment.

> **Culinary Use** <

Bran lies in the outer layers of the wheat kernel. When white flour is made, the mills separate the bran and wheatgerm and remove 35 per cent of the surface endosperm.

Quite the simplest way to put bran on the daily menu is to buy or make wholemeal bread. This does mean looking out for the words '100 per cent wholemeal', since some bread is sold as 81 or 85 per cent extraction, which means that the aleurone layer and bran have been removed.

Often bread is made with white flour and 'enriched' with bran; the natural product is preferable. Some people go to the trouble of buying stoneground wholemeal bread. The theory is that modern steel or roller plate mills reach such high speeds that the generated heat affects the quality of the flour and causes it to go rancid more quickly.

Natural wholemeal bread does not last so well as treated white bread, but can be kept in the refrigerator.

Whole wheat grains will also give you the benefit of bran. Cracked wheat is popular in American cookery as breakfast cereals, frumenty and pilaf.

In Eastern countries, wheat grains, known as *bulgur*, are boiled and partially cooked and made into delicious meatballs or sprinkled over salads. *Bulgur* and cracked wheat can be interchanged in any recipe.

The 'bran is beautiful' saga has even reached long, white spaghetti strands and transformed them into a splendid brown.

Firms making whole wheat pasta are making a fortune selling bran-rich macaroni, lasagne, vermicelli and spaghetti.

Bran itself can be bought as a ready-to-eat cereal, but the latest medical research tells us that it is much more effective in a natural, unprocessed form. Bran flakes or powder are widely available now from supermarkets as well as specialist stores. If it has not been treated with a stabilizer, natural bran can go rancid quickly and should be kept under refrigeration.

Natural bran powder or flakes can be added to daily cooking in many ways (but remember that more than a dessertspoon each is not needed unless prescribed by your doctor):

Stir into soups, especially thick or cream soups.

Mix into raw meat for hamburgers, meat loaves and mince mixtures.

Sprinkle over basic crumbles, and add to pastry mixes.

Stir into the bottom (not the top) of any breakfast cereal.

Sprinkle over stewed fruit before adding yogurt.

Add to casseroles instead of a thickener.

Use wholemeal flour to bake bread and add extra bran with extra liquid.

Make delicious bran muffins and bran biscuits to wean your family's tastebuds off refined foods.

> CABBAGE <

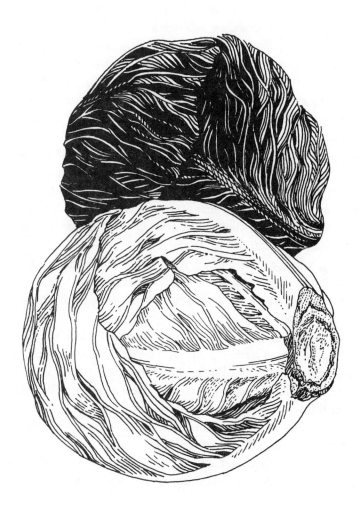

In América today, extract of cabbage is successfully being used to treat alcoholism. On hearing this, a historian surprised the doctors concerned by recalling that centuries ago the Roman Cato had advocated that anyone wishing to drink well at a banquet should first of all eat cabbage which had been dipped in vinegar. This, Cato believed, would allow the diner to enjoy his drink without suffering ill-effects, and what was more, prevent him from drinking too much.

Dr Roger Williams, the discoverer of pantothenic acid, was among the first to realize that some ordinary foods help in the fight against alcoholism. American Chemical Society bio-chemistry award winner, Dr William Shrive, has reported that he used a common amino acid found in cabbage juice, 'with good results' in the treatment of alcoholism.

During the 1970s groups of researchers at Texas University worked with alcoholic patients who wanted to give up drinking. First of all, the volunteers' diets were heavily supplemented with vitamins. These included magnesium with calcium; B vitamins high in inositol and cholin; Vitamin C with pantothenic acid; and capsules of vitamins A, D and E.

Then, white cabbage heads were extracted by filtration, and the white powder obtained was fed to the patients two or three times a day. The cabbage extracts were also supplemented with cabbage juices.

Within a short time the researchers noticed a marked change in the disposition of the patients. The irritability, quarrels and jumpiness so common during the withdrawal period decreased dramatically. One expert on alcoholism remarked on the absence of fist fights among the cabbage test volunteers.

As the experiment continued, almost half the patients reported that they had no difficulty in staying sober.

This initial success has been repeated in several centres through-out the U.S.A. A group working at the University of California at Berkeley found that a higher success rate was achieved if the patients were 'weaned' off alcohol with cabbage and vitamin therapy, then supported with psychotherapy and Alcoholics Anonymous. Other alternatives such as biofeedback, encounter groups and hypnotherapy are currently being used alongside cabbage treatments for alcoholics.

It should be said that prolonged medicinal use of concentrated cabbage extracts is not advisable, since this can interfere with the iodine absorption by the body.

Cabbage has another remarkable benefit. Tests in America and the U.S.S.R. have shown that cabbage juice and powder extract can heal stomach ulcers, especially the peptic variety, more quickly than powerful modern drugs.

In Moscow in 1964 the doctors Trusov and Belosludtsev treated fifty-five patients suffering from ulcers and chronic gastritis with dried juices from white cabbage. They reported that in every case there was some improvement, and 90 per cent of the ulcer patients healed quickly without further medicine.

In America, Dr L. R. Cheney gave raw cabbage juice to a hundred ulcer patients. Only five failed to show an improvement. Dr Cheney noticed that with the other patients the ulcer pain went in an average of five days and that the healing process was well under way by the fourteenth day.

This extraordinary healing action in cabbage is sometimes called vitamin U or the anti-ulcer factor.

Cabbage also has natural anti-germ and certain antibiotic qualities. Folk medicine believes that these antibiotic properties are greatly increased in pickled cabbage or sauerkraut.

> **Constituents** <

Cabbage contains the glycoside glucobrassin, mustard oil, the enzyme myrosinase and an anti-ulcer factor.

It also provides reasonable amounts of fibre, calcium, iron, potassium, vitamin A, vitamin C, vitamin K, with traces of the B vitamins thiamine, riboflavin and niacin.

> History <

Pliny declared roundly that cabbage was the finest medicinal plant in Roman history. He recommended it to treat no less than eighty-seven ailments, including ulcers, bronchitis, pleurisy, rheumatism, neuralgia, poor sight, eczema, jaundice and bad dreams.

Cato also thought very highly of cabbage and was convinced it prevented people from ever becoming drunkards. He also believed that cabbage kept the stomach healthy and that those who ate regular amounts would never develop pot bellies. In Rome and Greece cabbage was revered as celery was in ancient Egypt.

Cabbage is native to the Mediterranean and was introduced to Britain by the Romans (the conquering legions would hardly leave their most important medicinal vegetable behind). Other members of the *Brassica oleracea* family include kale, collard, kohl-rabi, brussels sprouts, cauliflower and broccoli.

True cabbage has played an important part in the history of food. The Dutch navy used sauerkraut extensively as a preventative against scurvy. Captain Cook, ever mindful of his men's suffering from the dread disease, considered sauerkraut 'highly anti-scorbutic' and ordered every man to be served with one pound of pickled cabbage twice a week.

The old English word for cabbage was 'colewort', and the present-day American term 'collard' is a corruption of this. Cole comes from the Latin *caulis*, stem.

In previous centuries cooks took a good deal more care with their cabbage than many of us do today. Medieval instructions for cooking shredded worts in butter sound strangely familiar to those interested in health food cookery. 'Take a large quantity of the worts – and shred them, and put butter or oyl thereto, and seethe them and serve forth – and let nothing else come nigh them.' In other words, classic conservation vegetable cooking.

The cabbage as we know it was introduced from Holland by Sir Arthur Ashley of Wilburg St Giles in Dorsetshire, and his monument in the local church has a fine carving of a cabbage on it. This improved continental cabbage is the one that settlers took with them to the new worlds of America and Australia.

> **Folk Use** <

In folk medicine cabbage is known as 'the doctor of the poor', a prince among the plants that heal.

Cabbage leaves are used as an instant first aid. The anti-inflammatory and germ-killing properties have always been valued in folk usage. In the days before sterilized bandages, cabbage leaves were used to bind up wounds, sores, boils and abscesses. Any cut, sore or lesion was treated in this way. Crushed cabbage leaves were promptly put on insect bites or stings and rubbed over pimples.

A favourite trick, still greatly popular in country districts, is to slip a hot cabbage leaf over any painful area. This is a treasured remedy in the case of rheumatism or arthritis and muscular aches and pains. Take a large cabbage leaf, cut out the central rib and heat it either by pouring on boiling water for a few minutes, or by ironing with an electric iron until it is as soft as velvet. You can even drape a cabbage leaf over a central heating radiator to warm it up. Naturally, this quick method is used only on intact skin, never where there are cuts or sores, in which case cabbage heated in boiling water would be more appropriate. Another good idea is to soak cabbage leaf in olive oil for one hour. The oil softens the leaf and makes it stick better.

In Ireland, hot cabbage leaves are wrapped around a severe sore throat and the raw juice sipped with honey. Hot compresses of cabbage are widely used in France today. They are made from cabbage leaves chopped finely, plunged in boiling water, then wrapped in clean muslin and applied to any painful area, especially to relieve period pains, stomach pains and liver attacks. For colds and asthma the hot compresses are placed on the chest. Like Pliny, folk tradition believes that cabbage is good for preventing nightmares. Cabbage water is drunk in the evening with a small pinch of sage.

Folk medicine believes that sauerkraut has its own very special antibiotic properties. Sauerkraut means quite literally sour cabbage, and it is fermented by *lactobacillus* which converts the sugar into lactic acid, which is responsible for the sour taste. This process preserves many of cabbage's active enzymes. Sauerkraut is used in Germany and many eastern European countries in very much the same way as yogurt, that is, to keep disease away and to promote youthful vigour.

> **Herbal Medicine** <

Juice from the winter cabbage is a herbal treatment for peptic ulcers. The juice must be freshly prepared each day and is never taken on an empty stomach. Short courses of cabbage juice are recommended too, for those with weak or over-acid stomachs. Cut up a fresh head of cabbage and extract the juice, adding a little water for taste. Between half and one litre of cabbage juice is taken in small amounts throughout each day, preferably after meals. A standard course of this therapy lasts three or four weeks.

Herbalists make use of cabbage's anti-inflammatory and germ-killing qualities to treat infections of the stomach and bowel. Cabbage juice or cabbage water is used in these cases. Slow healing wounds are treated with juice therapy and applications of leaves heated in boiling water.

Many herbalists, notably in Europe, are strong advocates of cabbage as a pain reliever, especially for rheumatism and arthritis. Short periodic courses of juice are recommended for people who suffer with these painful ailments. There is still, also, enthusiastic support for the good old-fashioned hot cabbage compress or poultice applied directly to a really painful joint.

Throughout the ages, cabbage juice or pickle has been used to treat and prevent drunkenness. John Evelyn and many other early herbalists refer to cabbage and ivy as the two prime medicines for people with drink problems.

An old herbal *lohoch* (medicine) was used for centuries for the 'after effects of a drunken orgie', to prevent the worse effects of too much alcohol. An old recipe for the *lohoch* indicates that a pinch of saffron be mixed with half a pound of honey and stirred into the juice of a pound of coleworts (white cabbage heads).

> **Culinary Use** <

The American writer Walter H. Page was a great Anglophile but he declared: 'The English have only three vegetables and two of them are cabbage.' Certainly, the horrid smell of over-cooked cabbage brings back vivid memories of school lunches to many British people.

Cabbage is perhaps the most under-rated and abused of all vegetables. It should be short-cooked to keep its crispness and to preserve the truly excellent health-giving active constituents.

When you cook cabbage there should be nothing more than a mild, appetizing smell. In fact, a ghastly smell when cooking indicates that the cabbage is being cooked at too high a temperature. What happens is this: cabbage is rich in volatile sulphur compounds. If cooking is too long or too hot these volatile compounds start to break down and escape, causing the distinctive over-cooked cabbage smell.

When the sulphur elements do break down during cooking they cause another uncomfortable reaction. During the digestive process in the stomach they cause gas or wind to form, resulting in discomfort and embarrassing noises.

Cabbage, with a rare medicine chest of goodness to offer, is found guilty without trial of causing offensive flatulence. Short cooking can prevent all this. Experiments have shown that practically no sulphur compounds break down when vegetables are cooked for eight to ten minutes at temperatures below boiling point. It is also a good idea to keep cabbage chilled or refrigerated to stop enzyme action breaking down the compounds.

Those with really susceptible digestions might try cooking cabbage in milk. This has the advantage of making sure that the temperature is kept low. Stainless steel steamers that fit neatly inside saucepans are good at reducing the temperatures as well.

Let us forget for the moment about boiled cabbage, however superbly cooked, and think of those countries which use this vegetable in a wide variety of imaginative ways.

This is certainly true of the Soviet Union. Indeed, a traditional Russian saying, roughly translated, means: 'Our food is the cabbage and the buckwheat.' In the U.S.S.R cabbage is made into the most delicious soups (known as *schi*) with meat stock, potato, onion, celery, turnip, bayleaf, tomato purée and the optional addition of spinach, young nettles or sauerkraut. In the eighteenth century the Empress Elizabeth shocked her French chef by insisting on *schi* being included not only on the daily menu but also in state banquets.

In Middle Eastern cooking, cabbage leaves are rolled into neat little cigar shapes stuffed with a variety of delicious mixtures such as lean lamb, rice and cinnamon or chick peas, rice, tomatoes, onions and allspice. Often the stuffed leaves are covered with a rich tomato or lemon sauce and left to bake very slowly in a moderate oven.

In French cooking, the heart is scooped out of a large firm white or green head of cabbage and replaced with fine pork stuffing. The cabbage is wrapped up in thin strips of bacon, then tied up in a cloth and fastened with string. It is braised very slowly for one and a half hours in a pan with bacon skin and slices of onion and carrot. Then the magnificent head is presented at the table.

Michel Guérard invented a low calorie cabbage pie with onion and herb stuffing for his *cuisine minceur*. In Scandinavian cooking, red cabbage is sliced very thinly and mixed with slices of eating apples, finely chopped onion and a few sprinklings of nutmeg, cayenne, or caraway. The cabbage is then cooked in a minute amount of water with butter or oil in a tightly lidded pan. Just before the cabbage is tender a few tablespoons of vinegar are added.

In Germany, small frauleins learn to make sauerkraut at their mother's knee. It is quite easy. A large firm head of white cabbage is shredded finely into an earthenware crock. It is arranged in layers about one inch thick and a teaspoon of sea salt sprinkled over each layer with a few caraway seeds and juniper berries. When the crock is full of these alternate layers a plate is firmly placed on top and the pressure kept up by adding a heavy weight. Ideally the plate should not quite cover the top of the crock to allow the scum to rise up over the sides and be scooped off daily. The sauerkraut is kept in a warm place to encourage the lactic fermentation. When the foam or bubbling has stopped, usually after four or five weeks, the sauerkraut is transferred to sterilized jars with sealed lids and stored in a cool place for use as needed.

Raw cabbage, of course, is a fine way of getting the best nutritional and medicinal values of this vegetable. The nicest way of eating raw cabbage is in the form of coleslaw. A most delicious coleslaw can be made by mixing the three main varieties of cabbage together, using equal amounts of red, white and green cabbage. Shred the heads, finely or chunkily according to your own taste, into a large bowl, add chopped watercress, chopped crisp dessert apple, a crushed clove of garlic, black pepper and a lemon juice and olive oil dressing. Stir well and add a carton of sour cream or yogurt.

A yogurt and vinegar dressing goes well with coleslaw. Caraway seeds have a particular affinity with cabbage, and will not only add spice and bite to a raw dish but also give their valuable carminative property. The Americans make a delicious coleslaw with shredded green cabbage, diced pineapple, apple and banana, about six fresh mint leaves, a few fresh basil leaves if they are available, and a handful of peanuts, with mayonnaise or Thousand Island dressing. Another alternative is to use shredded green or purple cabbage, chopped green pepper, chopped pimento, grated onion, chives and chopped dill pickle mixed with mayonnaise or yogurt dressing.

> CARAWAY <

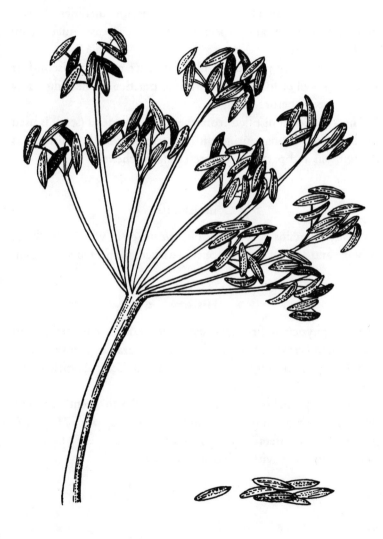

> Health <

Caraway seed is one of the major carminative herbs with the strength to relieve flatulence or wind and ease the griping pains they cause. Caraway has a marked action in preventing excessive intestinal wind forming so it is obviously a good thing to take before heavy meals. It is also a digestion stimulant, and like dill has the nice quality of bringing warmth and comfort to the stomach. Caraway also has its own specific qualities. It is a natural disinfectant and expectorant which can ease mucus from the bronchial tubes.

People who are prey to regular flatulence or gassy discomfort would do well to follow the European practice of chewing a few caraway seeds before eating.

The volatile oil distilled from the dried, ripe fruit (seed) is used medicinally as a flavouring and a carminative. Its constituents are unusual and particularly interesting to chemists.

> Constituents <

Caraway contains a volatile oil, *oleum cari*, which produces carvone and a derivative, limonene; a fixed oil, proteins and resin.

> History <

Arabian physicians first used caraway seeds as a medicine and called them *karawya*. Dioscorides thought caraway seeds brought a healthy pink colour to the cheeks and advised pale girls to eat them.

Caraway probably came to Europe in the thirteenth century where it became immensely popular. In Shakespeare's *Henry IV*, Justice Shallow offers Sir John Falstaff ' . . . a last year's pippin of my own graffing with a dish of caraway'.

> Folk Use <

Caraway seeds are an instant folk aid to getting rid of painful stomach wind. It is common practice, especially in Austria and Germany, to chew a few seeds until relief is obtained. Another standard practice is to drink caraway tea made from the bruised and crushed seeds, and sip it warm or cold whenever needed, using half to one teaspoon per cup.

Stronger caraway teas are used to promote menses and stimulate milk in breast-feeding mothers.

Folk medicine believes caraway is good for all the organs of digestion, and that it 'sweetens' the bowel.

For many centuries in England caraway seeds enjoyed a vogue as a treatment for hysterical ladies. Angry or choleric men who lost their tempers easily were urged to take a cup of caraway tea, no doubt on the principle that such strong emotion was very bad for the digestion.

The American Indians made an embrocation of caraway leaves steeped in buffalo oil for braves with stiff muscles.

In the countries where caraway is much valued it is generously used in the regional cookery.

> Herbal Medicine <

Oil or spirit of caraway is used in many herbal medicines to treat flatulent indigestion. Where this is habitual or of long standing, alternative medicine prefers to get to the root of the problem to find if it's emotional or physical, and treat it carefully. On the dietary side, caraway seeds chewed before a meal are medically acknowledged as a good preventative. They are also helpful in stimulating the gastric juices. Caraway tea can be taken in the same way before meals, or given to small children in teaspoon doses.

To stimulate sluggish appetites and digestions, crush half a teaspoon of caraway seeds to a smooth paste with a little water, dilute and drink about twenty minutes before meals.

Because of its carminative and disinfectant properties, caraway is also used in certain cases of diarrhoea.

> **Culinary Use** <

Caraway seed is lovingly used in German and Austrian cookery. It is sprinkled onto cakes, soups and cheeses, and of course is the flavour in delicious fragrant caraway bread. In Scandinavia, polenta-type rye bread is cooked with caraway seeds and makes an excellent basis for *smörgåsbord* and sandwiches.

In Europe, caraway is coated with sugar to make 'sugar plums', a popular digestive or dessert. It is also the flavouring of the liqueur kümmel, and certain kinds of schnapps.

Caraway seed used to be very popular in English cookery, especially in Elizabethan times, but has rather lost ground in the last century. The seeds used to be served with hot roast apples (Shakespeare's pippins) and put into seed cakes.

In Hungary and Czechoslovakia, caraway seeds are used in many meat dishes, especially roast pork, and in some goulashes. Throughout Europe, caraway leaves are used fresh in salads, where their milder flavour blends well with other ingredients.

It is intriguing to note that caraway has a particular affinity with cabbage, a notoriously 'windy' vegetable. Sprinkle a few caraway seeds into the cabbage before boiling, and you will be surprised at the nutty, unusual flavour.

> CELERY <

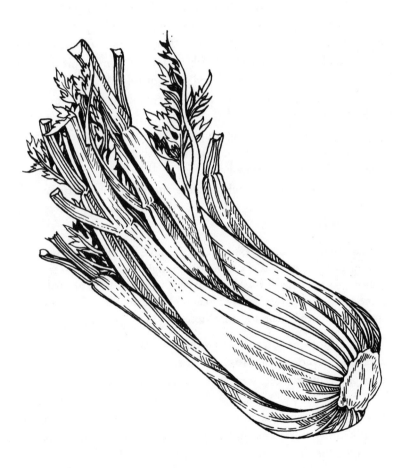

Celery is one of the great tonics among the plants that heal. Ancient doctors in Egypt and Greece valued celery highly and used it as a medicine to treat illnesses ranging from strained nerves to aching joints.

In Europe, especially Britain, celery seed tea is traditionally the great classic folk medicine for arthritis and aching joints.

This folk treatment prompted the research by Dr David Lewis and his team at Aston University in Birmingham. Dr Lewis went to his local supermarket and bought as many bunches of ordinary celery as he could carry. Back at the laboratory the celery stalks were extracted with water by homogenizing and filtration. The powder obtained was dissolved and subjected, first of all on rats, to the standard pharmaceutical tests for anti-arthritic drugs.

First results were so encouraging that a whole series of controlled tests began. These confirmed that celery has a definite, beneficial effect on arthritis.

What defied the researchers were the precise constitutents in celery which had such marked anti-inflammatory effects. Dr Lewis writes:

It was found that celery extract contained an anti-inflammatory substance, or substances. Work is now in progress to identify these substances. So far a sterol of the stigmasterol class has been isolated with some anti-inflammatory action. It seems likely that other substances with stronger activity remain to be isolated.

This is not uncommon in natural medicine. Celery has caused a reaction among scientists and doctors very similar to that of papaya: 'It works but we don't yet know exactly how.'

What is known is that the anti-inflammatory agent in celery can break down uric acid in painful joints and help synovial fluid to flow more smoothly again. No doubt this action partly accounts for the stimulating effect that celery has as a food.

Interestingly enough, celery is an excellent food for slimmers.

Not only for its low calorie count (one large raw stalk has five calories), but also because it appeases a hungry appetite. Chew a celery stalk slowly before meals, or mix half a teaspoon of honey in a glass of celery juice and sip slowly to reduce hunger pangs very effectively.

Modern research has discovered that all parts of the celery plant – stalks, leaves, roots and seeds – contain the medicinally active principles.

Celery stalks contain their share of the anti-inflammatory principle, as Dr Lewis's research showed. However, other tests have shown that celery seeds and leaves contain the most powerful concentration of the known active agents. So granny, sipping her celery seed tea for arthritic relief, showed great instinctive wisdom.

Celery is one of those foods which baffles modern technology because it has apparent contradictory actions. On the one hand, it has proven stimulant, tonic qualities; on the other, it is used for its calming effect on the nerves. Folk users find this natural and not unusual. Ginseng is another such food which tones up the whole system and yet effectively relaxes as well. It is fascinating to note that both these foods, ginseng and celery, are highly valued in the East and the West for their use as a traditional aphrodisiac.

Celery has a most individual combination of active ingredients. It is unusual to find volatile oils and a natural hormone in one plant. It is these powerful constituents acting together in one vegetable which make celery such an outstanding tonic and stimulant.

> Constituents <

Celery contains a volatile oil including terpenes and phenols, apiol, resins, saponin and a natural hormone.

It also provides moderate amounts of fibre, iron, calcium, phosphorus, potassium, vitamin C and the B vitamin, niacin..

> History <

The *Apium graveolens* plant originated in the Levant and spread gradually to southern Europe. The Roman legions took celery with them to Britain as a medicine, but it was then a small, bitter herb whose leaves tasted like lovage. The colder, damp climate suited celery and it grew taller and less bitter.

Celery became popular in Europe first as a herb or medicinal plant and then as a food. Even so, the first recorded use of celery as a food plant was in France in 1623.

Italian horticulturists were originally responsible for breeding out the bitterness of celery and producing a crisp, delicious stalk. They also developed another variety of *Apium graveolens* for its swollen, turnip-shaped root, which is known as celeriac.

The earliest crops had to be blanched or earthed up with soil, paper or boards both to protect them against frost and to improve the taste. Blanched celery is usually creamy white in colour.

Farmers in Florida, U.S.A. revolutionized commercial practice by producing green, self-blanching celery. This variety is now universally popular because it tastes so good and is easier to produce. It also has the advantage of containing chlorophyll as well. The U.S.A. is now the largest producer of celery in the world.

> Folk Use <

Did woman know what celery
bestows upon a man,
she would go forth to search for it
from Rome to Turkestan.

This lovely old anonymous bit of doggerel more than hints at celery's reputed powers as an aphrodisiac. Legend also has it that celery was the ingredient in the love potion that had such dramatic effect on Tristan and Isolde.

Before this is dismissed as picturesque fantasy, it might be well to remember that the British 'old wives' who were so magnificently vindicated by their use of celery seed tea in arthritis also used it to treat worn out or sexually impotent men.

Traditional uses of celery to treat arthritis and rheumatism started in ancient Egypt, where doctors prescribed seeds, leaves and stalks to patients suffering from these disorders. They also prescribed ground celery seeds dissolved in wine for those suffering from nervous complaints and the mysterious illness âaâ, which modern scholars have identified as depression.

The Greeks were accurate observers of the tonic powers of celery. When supplies were short it was rationed and fed to the most needy. Athletes, for instance, were often awarded celery for their sporting achievements. It was so valued that a colloquial phrase went into the language: 'He's on his last legs, give him celery.' The Greeks expressed the juice from raw celery with stones and drank it before meals as a tonic.

In Russia, a well-known traditional nerve tonic is made from finely chopped celery stalks and leaves and hot cider vinegar. The mixture is kept tightly covered and taken in teaspoon doses three times a day.

Celery juice is a Hungarian gipsy remedy for blemished skin. The Romanies give themselves seven-day courses of stewed celery dishes for rheumatism, arthritis and to reduce high blood pressure.

In Europe and America celery is traditionally taken after debilitating illnesses, especially flu, to beat the depressed feeling that sometimes follows and to speed toxins from the system.

> **Herbal Medicine** <

Herbalists make good use of the entire celery plant in their medicines. An infusion of celery leaves is considered an excellent remedy for pulmonary or stubborn catarrh, such as in bronchitis. A decoction of the root is used against gravel and jaundice. Celery root boiled into a broth with milk is regarded as an excellent remedy in gout or rheumatism but is not used in cases of nephritis. Root medicine is sweetened and made into lozenges which are effective against irritating coughs.

A fluid extract of the seeds is made as a tonic and five or ten drops are taken in hot water three times a day before meals.

Celery seed tea (one teaspoon of crushed or bruised seeds to one cup of boiling water) is a standard remedy in all cases of arthritis, rheumatism, fibrositis and aching joints.

The American herbalist, Jethro Kloss, is an advocate of celery juice used regularly to maintain a good pure complexion.

> Homeopathic Medicine <

Homeopathic chemists isolate the apiol in celery and parsley and use it both to treat and to prevent certain types of colds and catarrh. Homeopaths, like herbalists, strongly recommend apiol and celery itself to all arthritic patients.

Apiol is still used in the East to treat malaria.

> Culinary Use <

A bit of common sense in the kitchen can bring the benefits of the latest research straight into daily life.

The indications are that the anti-inflammatory agent in celery is mildly soluble in cold water and highly soluble in hot water. Lengthy boiling will destroy other active ingredients.

Clearly, raw fresh celery and celery seed decoctions are going to provide the most benefits.

Luckily, celery is such a crunchy delicious vegetable that it is a pleasure to take it as a 'medicine'. Use imagination to add celery to many salads and *hors d'oeuvre*, and, of course, never throw the leaves away. Use them in salads too, or chop finely and sprinkle on dishes with parsley.

Liven up celery sticks by stuffing them with hummus, or dipping them into a remoulade sauce with parsley, gherkins and tarragon.

Edwardian chefs used raw celery most imaginatively in their

grand banquets. Celery pieces were sprinkled with lemon juice, dressed with a pimento mayonnaise and arranged in orange or grapefruit halves.

Cooked celery can retain some of its fine values if approached in these ways. Braise it slowly, as the French do, in a minute amount of water or meat stock on a low heat. Add celery to your basic soup stocks or casseroles but reserve a few leaves and finely chopped stalks to add several minutes before serving.

Celery seed with the concentrated goodness of the plant is obviously something to get to know and use regularly. Celery seed tea is quite palatable and easy to make. A standard brew is made with one teaspoon of bruised or crushed seeds to about one cup of boiling water. Allow to stand for approximately four minutes, strain and sweeten to taste. If this is unpalatable at first, add the crushed seeds to your regular Indian or Chinese brew.

Our worthy Victorian ancestors had a superb way of using celery seed and all its medicinal values. Quite simply, they soaked celery seed in brandy for about two weeks. Victorian ladies instructed their cooks to make this 'celery essence' without realizing that they were preparing a classic herbal tincture, in which the volatile and active constituents of celery dissolve into the alcohol and are preserved.

A recipe of 1870 takes one tablespoon of celery seed to 200ml of brandy. The seeds are steeped in the brandy for a few weeks and then strained out and the mixture carefully stored and used a few drops at a time for soups, stews, sauces and casseroles. A small phial of the celery essence was added to the medicine cabinet and used for the emergencies of Victorian life, such as fainting, ladies with fits of the vapours, or gentlemen who were rather too lethargic.

Celery seed is widely available from health food stores or specialist shops and can be ground up in ordinary pepper grinders for use as salt. You can, of course, buy ready-made celery salt and use it in every instance instead of ordinary salt, only more lavishly.

> CHICORY <

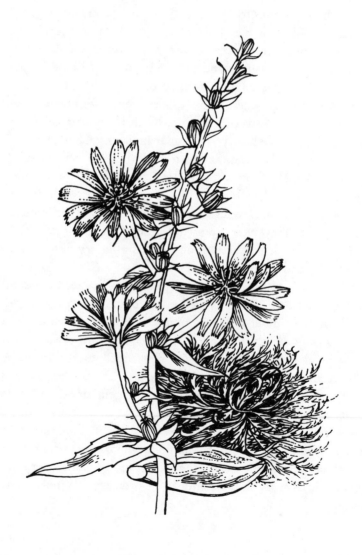

> Health <

The *Cichorium* family gives us a herb, chicory, and two closely related delicate vegetables, chicory and endive. Vegetable chicory is also known as French endive but endive itself is the correct name for another species in the same family.

All members of the chicory family share the same active principles, but the vegetables contain much less than the roots. The whole plant acts beneficially on the liver and is valued for this effect in alternative medicine, where it is used to treat jaundice, gallstones and many liver disorders. Chicory acts as a mild stimulant for bile production and is considered to have a cleansing effect on the whole system. This vegetable is also a digestive aid. It does not act dramatically on stomach wind like caraway or dill, but generally tones and improves the whole digestion, making a valuable long-term ally against indigestion.

Herb chicory, still known as succory by country people, is a familiar wild flower with its exquisite blue star-like petals because it will obligingly grow almost anywhere, an indestructible wayside companion. The long tap root of this flower is widely cultivated commercially for its use as the popular coffee substitute, chicory coffee. The roots are carefully washed and dried, then roasted and ground to make herb coffee or coffee bean and chicory mixtures.

Chicory coffee and chicory vegetables are known in European tradition as an aid to slimmers. No doubt this has something to do with the cleansing effect of the plant, but also owes something to the fact that well roasted chicory coffee helps to fight that empty feeling.

> Constituents <

Chicory and endive vegetables contain a bitter principle, vitamin A, potassium, moderate amounts of fibre, iron, calcium and niacin.

Chicory herb root contains a bitter principle, intybin and inulin.

> History <

The Romans ate endive as a salad and a vegetable and used succory as a herb. Chicory was one of the most popular vegetables in Arabian cooking, as its slightly bitter taste balanced more exotic flavours.

As the coffee-drinking craze began to spread across Europe, chicory gradually became more cultivated and gardeners began to experiment with varieties and improve them with blanching.

Linnaeus, the great Swedish botanist, used chicory flowers in his floral clock at Upsala. The flower heads have the extraordinary habit of opening and closing at precise hours throughout the season, like a small clockwork machine.

> Folk Use <

Galen called chicory 'the friend of the liver', and folk medicine certainly agrees with that. During liver troubles every part of the plant is used in medicines and masses of vegetable chicory or endive is eaten raw in salads. In France, chicory is considered a vital food to eat during jaundice.

In country tradition, chicory is valued as a depurative, with the power to cleanse the system of toxins. Chicory juice from the root and vegetable leaves is one of the great folk spring cleansers. It is believed to get winter out of the system and purify the blood. The concentrated juice is a powerful medicine and, like all natural spring cleansers, is only taken for about two weeks once a year.

According to legend, the endive plant grew from the tears of a French girl who waited for her lover's ship to return. For centuries endive seeds were an important constituent in love philtres.

Folk medicine has it that chicory is added to coffee not so much for cheapness, but mainly because it counteracts any irritating effect of caffein.

❯ Herbal Medicine ❮

The old herbalists thought highly of chicory. Parkinson declared it to be 'a fine, cleansing, jovial plant'.

Today, chicory is used in herbal medicines to treat liver complaints, jaundice, gout, rheumatism and some kidney disorders. In the days before antibiotics it was a popular specific against tuberculosis.

To prevent or treat gallstones a tea is made from the shredded root or dried leaves of chicory. Boil two teaspoons of shredded root in one cup of water for three minutes. Allow to stand, covered, for 10 minutes. Take one cup daily for about one week. If the dried leaf is used it need only be brought to the boil and infused for 15 minutes. Chicory remedies are tonic, mildly laxative and diuretic.

❯ Culinary Use ❮

The chicory or endive (sometimes called escarole in the U.S.A.) that we buy as a vegetable has been blanched in the dark to take away some of its natural bitterness. Nonetheless chicory leaves give to salads that touch of bitterness which adds another dimension. Some chefs believe that chicory is less bitter if it is not cut with a knife.

Herb chicory coffee is made quite easily, in much the same way as dandelion root coffee, by gentle roasting and grinding. Many a thrifty housewife has stretched her coffee beans out by mixing them with a few spoonfuls of roast chicory.

Small, tight heads of chicory make a good cooked vegetable. They can be boiled with a dash of lemon juice, or braised in the oven with butter or vegetable oil and then served with bechamel or cheese sauce.

In Europe chicory or endive stumps are known as *gourilos*. French cooks would not dream of throwing the stumps away; they use them as a vegetable in their own right or serve them cooked as an *hors d'oeuvre*.

> DILL <

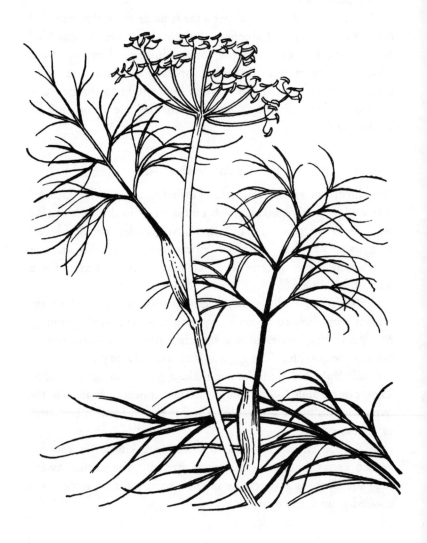

> Health <

There can be few windy babies who have not had their 'burpulence' relieved by this kindly herb. Mothers everywhere bless 'gripe water', as dill medicine is popularly known. Chemists use the dried, ripe fruit with its rich component of volatile oil to make dill water, which is so soothing to gassy stomachs.

The British Pharmaceutical Codex gives a prescription for dill water with this comment: 'Dill water is a carminative used in the treatment of flatulence in infants.'

Windy adults, too, would do well to treat their flatulence with dill water, as it is so relieving and mild to sensitive digestions. One of dill's pleasant qualities is the warm, comforting feeling it gives to the stomach. No doubt this contributes to its long-standing success with crotchety babies, especially at night time.

> Constituents <

The chief constituent is the volatile oil *oleum anethi* which, like caraway, contains carvone.

> History <

Dill has a long history as a kindly herb. Its name comes from the Norse *dilla*, meaning to lull or soothe, and many ancient cultures valued these qualities. So powerful was dill considered to be that by the Middle Ages it was one of the special herbs used against evil.

In *Nymphidia* Drayton wrote:

> Therewith her Vervain and her Dill
> that hinderith Witches of their Will.

During the great religious revival of John Wesley, dill became nicknamed the 'meeting house seed'. Evangelical sermons were fiery and often four or five hours long. The congregation chewed dill seed to stay hunger pangs and stop their stomachs from rumbling, or making other impolite noises.

> Folk Use <

Dill is cherished as a lullaby remedy, not only for fractious babies, but also dyspeptic adults.

The ancient Egyptians used dill tea to treat turbulent, gassy stomachs and this remedy has come right down to us today.

A common recipe for dill tea uses one teaspoon of ripe seeds to one litre of water. Add the crushed seeds to the boiling water, strain and sweeten to taste. This is traditionally used for hiccoughs as well.

Dill, a native of the Mediterranean, grows wild in many European countries and especially in the Soviet Union. Soviet mothers neatly combine the milk-stimulating and soothing qualities of dill tea by drinking a cup just before breast feeding their babies. A natural preventative measure if ever there was one.

> Herbal Medicine <

The whole dill plant is considered soothing to the nervous system.

Herbalists also make use of dill leaves in medicines. As well as combating flatulence, the leaves are slightly anti-spasmodic and also stimulate the gastric juices.

Dill leaves and seed are recommended for regular use by nursing mothers, especially just after the baby has been born. In Europe, the leaves are boiled in milk or water as a remedy for colic-type stomach upsets and sleeplessness.

Nicholas Culpeper, as usual, expressed his opinion pungently:

The seed is of more use than the leaves, and more effectual to digest raw and vicious humours, and is used in medicines that serve to expel wind, and the pains preceding therefrom . . .

> Culinary Use <

Dill has an affinity with sour or pickled dishes and is well known in combination with pickled cucumbers or gherkins. In the

U.S.A. and Australia these are known as dill pickles. They are soured, like sauerkraut, by lactic fermentation, and contain the carminative (or wind-expelling) qualities *par excellence*. In fact, in Australia, the word dill applied to a person is a typically robust insult.

Dill is a favourite herb for Scandinavians, who use it in fish dishes very much as the French use *court bouillon*. To poach fish, water is brought to the boil and flavoured with dill leaves. It is an especially popular method for cooking salmon. Fresh or dried leaves are sprinkled generously over summer salads for a distinctive flavour.

In British cooking, dill sauce is an old favourite with mutton. A few crushed seeds are added to cabbage or cauliflower when it is cooking, in much the same way as caraway. A sprinkling of dill seed in any kind of apple pie makes a delicious mixture.

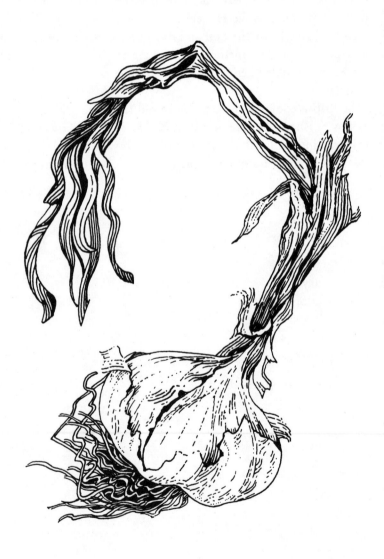

Garlic, like its cousin, onion, has a remarkable effect on the heart. There is sound scientific evidence to support the theory that regular use of garlic can prevent heart attacks.

Also, there is a widespread folk belief that daily garlic can help to prevent cancer. It is said that in France the incidence of both cancer and heart attacks are lowest where the consumption of garlic is highest. A similar theory is applied to Bulgaria. In the U.S.S.R. today, extracts of garlic are being used as part of the treatment for skin cancer.

India presents a clear picture because in certain definable areas the people will not eat onions or garlic for religious reasons. Heart attacks in these communities are more common than in those which make lavish use of garlic and onions. Obviously this geographical profile is one reason why Indian doctors have led the world research into these two vegetables. Among their other observations, the doctors have found that in southern Madras women are always given garlic during the second half of their pregnancies. These women do not suffer from toxaemia, a complication of pregnancy accompanied by high blood pressure.

Veterinary practice, too, triggered off the intensive Indian research. Horses and other animals which develop clots or thrombosis are widely treated with garlic and onions throughout Europe. Indian tests showed that garlic had a serum-lowering effect and that it increased fibrinolysis, the ability of the body to dissolve the clots which can form inside veins or blood vessels. Other Indian tests showed that garlic lowered the concentration of sugar in the blood both of normal and diabetic patients.

Scientists at the University of Benghazi in Libya confirmed the Indian findings. They fed test animals oil of garlic in doses varying from 0.2 mg to 1.0 mg and noticed that the effects were in direct relation to the amounts. At the higher dosage, there was a 51 per cent reduction in atherosclerotic lesions and a 30 per cent reduction in serum cholesterol.

Quite clearly, garlic plays an important preventative role against heart and arterial disease and high blood pressure.

Garlic is also one of the most powerful natural antiseptics. In 1936 the Italian Dr G. Caspar first demonstrated that garlic can destroy *staphylococcus*. Then the Russian scientist T. Yanovich introduced garlic oil into colonies of bacteria. He reported that all movement of germs stopped within five minutes.

During lengthy experiments in Germany during the 1950s, Dr J. Klosa showed that the active oils in garlic can actually unite with a virus and make it inactive.

Folk medicine has always believed that garlic can increase resistance to infection, and modern research thoroughly vindicates the age-old uses.

From this picture, garlic emerges as a potent ally against disease, with many good reasons why we should use this pungent bulb in our daily life. Yet many people avoid garlic because it 'doesn't agree' with them or, more probably, because it makes the breath smell.

There is good reason to believe that the breath only smells offensively of garlic if the digestion is out of order. Garlic is actually an *aid* to good digestion. It stimulates the stomach secretions and the gall bladder and prevents putrefaction taking place in the stomach. Garlic's effectiveness against digestive troubles was confirmed by Dr Harry Barowsky and Dr L. J. Boyd. Writing in the *Review of Gastroenterology*, they describe their use of garlic capsules on fifty patients who suffered from 'various disorders commonly associated with gastro intestinal symptoms'. These conditions included indigestion, uncomfortable flatulence, distention, nausea and vomiting. Improvement among the patients was so marked that the doctors commented: 'This remedy should merit consideration in treatment when these symptoms . . . are present.'

Assuredly, any slight anti-social aspects of garlic are more than outweighed by its medicinal values. Garlic tends to detoxify the entire digestive system, with special influence on the heart, blood vessels and blood pressure. Raw garlic provides the most powerful benefits and can be introduced gradually into the diet in salads and grated vegetables. Remember that the good old folk tradition of chewing a sprig of parsley after garlicky meals does constitute an effective breath deodorizer.

> Constituents <

Garlic contains essential oil containing sulphur, allyl disulphide, allicin, alliin, vitamins A and C, and nicotinic acid.

> History <

The slaves toiling to build the great pyramids of Egypt were given a ration of garlic to keep them strong enough to lift the huge stones. One day the garlic failed to appear and the slaves downed tools in protest, causing the first recorded strike in history. The ancient Greeks valued the strengthening powers of garlic and fed it to their athletes and wrestlers in large quantities. However, to the Greeks, garlic was 'the stinking rose', beautiful but smelly, and no one was allowed to eat garlic for a few hours before entering the temples of Cybele, mother of the gods.

Homer tells us that when the villainous Circe was changing Ulysses' companions into a herd of pigs, Ulysses himself escaped this fate by quickly chewing a bulb of 'yellow garlic'.

The Roman army marched and conquered on a veritable wave of garlic since the bulb was dedicated to Mars, the god of war. The soldiers chewed cloves of garlic just before battle to make them brave, and army doctors rubbed garlic on wounds to stop sepsis and prescribed them for all chest and intestinal complaints among the legions. Pliny gives us one of his inimitable lengthy lists of ailments which garlic can treat, including colds, parasites and high blood pressure.

Dioscorides, Nero's personal physician, recommended garlic

for more peaceful uses. He mixed it with syrup made from honey to make a gargle to improve the voice, a practice still followed by operatic tenors in Italy today. One might speculate that Nero gargled with honey and garlic to sing to his fiddle while Rome burned.

Garlic's antiseptic powers were greatly valued in the Middle Ages during the terrible years of plague. According to popular history, French priests were able to visit the most stricken areas of London without catching the disease because they made medicinal use of garlic. In contrast, the non-garlic-eating English priests suffered appalling losses from plague.

In early centuries the English races had none of the nose-wrinkling attitude to garlic so common today. Chaucer wrote of his Sompnour: 'Wel loved he garlike, onions and lekes.'

Cole's *Art of Simpling* in the sixteenth century describes the barbarous sport of cock-fighting. He says that cocks fed garlic are 'most stout to fight and so are horses'.

In Europe today the old superstition persists that a runner chewing garlic in a race can somehow prevent anyone else getting ahead of him. Athletes have been known to plug garlic cloves firmly in their teeth during important competitions.

> Folk Use <

All the different countries which use garlic in traditional folk medicine are agreed on one thing: it is synonymous with vitality and long life.

An old Spanish proverb says: 'Where you find garlic you find good health.' In France, King Henri IV was baptized with a clove of garlic rubbed on his tongue, followed by a sip of armagnac. Some French parents still do this today, to prepare their children symbolically for the challenges of life.

Throughout the ages, folk users in England, America, France and Italy have mixed chopped garlic with honey or sugar to treat colds and influenza. Children with asthma or whooping cough have this mixture rubbed on their chests. Garlic syrup is still a popular remedy for chronic bronchitis or stubborn catarrh and is invaluable in breaking up a cold. Many country folk swore that the dreaded tuberculosis could be cured by raw garlic eaten every day.

The same garlic syrup was used by Dr Albert Schweitzer to reduce fevers at his jungle hospital in French Equatorial Africa.

There is a persistent folk belief that garlic is an anti-cancer agent, ranging from countries as different as Finland and Texas. The father of modern medicine, Hippocrates, mentions it for the treatment of certain tumours.

Folk uses of garlic throughout the ages were brought to a peak with a fine flourish by the Victorians. Doctors invaded the sick room with strong-smelling garlic lotions, potions and poultices. The eminent Dr Bowles advocated the application of a garlic poultice to the feet for those patients with weak stomachs who nevertheless needed the medicinal power of garlic during colds and fevers. Dr Bowles assured them that the garlic would go so quickly into the bloodstream that it could be smelt, delicately of course, on the breath the next morning. On a more basic level, farm labourers stuck cloves of garlic into their woolly socks to ward off flu and colds during the long winters. Many Victorian kitchens had a crock of garlic steeped in vinegar in the corner to treat septic sores and wounds.

The French make a delicious tincture of garlic by crushing the cloves in brandy. This is a valuable remedy for asthma, hoarseness, sore throats and disorders of the lungs and chest.

A strong smelling ointment is made by crushing cloves of garlic with lard and olive oil. This is known as Devil's Mustard and is rubbed or massaged on to painful rheumatic or arthritic joints or any sore sprains or aches. Garlic ointment acts as a decongestant on the lungs in cases of asthma, whooping cough and catarrh.

Alfred Franklin, in *La Vie d'autrefois*, says:

In the sixteenth century, the Parisians did not neglect to eat garlic with fresh butter during the month of May and were quite convinced that this rustic diet strengthened their health for the whole year.

In fact the practice of revitalizing the system with garlic in May is still widely popular in certain countries, ranging from France to Iceland.

Traditionally, garlic has held the same high reputation as yogurt for promoting long life and health. When Mrs Eleanor Roosevelt was in her eighties she was asked the secret of her remarkable memory. 'A clove of garlic every day,' she replied.

> Herbal Medicine <

Garlic is a very important herbal medicine and is one of the most powerful natural antiseptics known to the herbalist. Throughout alternative medicine, garlic is believed to give protection against all kinds of infectious ailments, including epidemic illnesses and parasites.

Garlic's actions are classified herbally as antiseptic, anti-toxic, vermifuge (kills worms and parasites), expectorant (relieves mucus), diuretic, digestive, diaphoretic (promotes perspiration) and tonic. This is a formidable list and one that is endorsed by *Martindale*, the official British Extra Pharmacopoeia. Herbalists utilize garlic's cholesterol-lowering potential in their medicines for patients suffering from heart conditions and high blood pressure. Garlic is believed to keep the arteries healthy generally, and is valued, for that reason, in all disorders of old age.

Garlic acts strongly on mucus membrane in all parts of the body, and herbalists use these expectorant qualities to treat bronchitis and chest colds. Raw garlic is used as a vermifuge to expel parasites, including tapeworm. The patient is advised to fast during the day and take several cloves of garlic at night. One garlic clove is covered with olive oil and used as a pessary.

Garlic is a specific remedy against whooping cough and asthma, obesity, rheumatism, arthritis and sciatica.

Garlic's volatile essential oils quickly penetrate the blood-stream. Herbalists recommend it as a regular tonic, preventative and antiseptic dietary aid.

As a herbal medicine garlic should be taken raw, but herbalists also prescribe garlic pearles which many people find more agreeable. Garlic pearles contain essential oil of garlic and were invented by Dr J. A. Höfel. The idea is that the garlic oil is mixed with vegetable oil and wrapped in a capsule to dissolve in the stomach without aftertaste or smell. The pearles preserve more of the essential oil than cooked cloves of garlic and are therefore very effective.

However, it is wise to remember that garlic oil is potent and that large or medicinal amounts should not be given to small children.

> **Culinary Use** <

Garlic is immensely popular in France, especially in Provence, where every dish is flavoured with garlic. It is the essential flavouring of the great soups, meat, fish and sauce dishes of *haute cuisine*. Just how much garlic goes into a dish is obviously a matter of personal taste, and can either be a faint flavouring or the dominant factor. Some French cooks use garlic lavishly, and what is more they get away with it. One writer described how he was given a dish of what he thought were chick peas in a little French country inn. Remarking on their unusually delicious flavour to the proprietor, he was told: 'But monsieur, those are garlic cloves braised in butter.'

The famous and beloved *aïoli* – or garlic and egg sauce – allows two large cloves of garlic for each person. *Aïoli garni* is a Friday dish as well as one of the traditional Christmas Eve dishes. *Aïoli* is served with potatoes, sweet peppers, various fish, hard-boiled eggs or chick peas, and is an inventive and surprisingly delicate addition to anyone's repertoire of recipes. Garlic soup itself is very popular throughout France. French children are practically brought up on bread rubbed with cloves of garlic and poured over with olive oil.

In Jewish cookery a strongly flavoured anchovy and garlic sauce is served with fried fish. This is called zemino sauce and we can use it equally well to add interest to winter salads.

Ideally, garlic should be pounded in a mortar and pestle or pressed through a garlic press. Chefs have a trick of laying the clove on its flat side then whanging it with the flat side of a broad knife. This enables the garlic to be minutely chopped and extracts the maximum of oil.

> GINSENG <

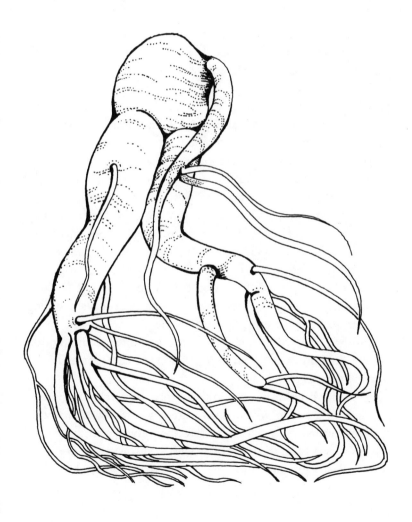

Ginseng is called 'the root of heaven' in China, where it has been valued as a medicine for over 2,000 years. Today, poorer people will work hours overtime or even take two jobs rather than go without their precious roots of ginseng.

This treasured root is believed in the East to have quite extraordinary powers. To the people, ginseng is their finest tonic, rejuvenator and aphrodisiac, a most essential aid to vibrant health and virility. A large body of doctors and scientists agree with this folk use, since ginseng is now official in the Japanese and Russian pharmacopoeias and has been recognized for centuries in the Chinese Materia Medica.

Doctors in those countries credit ginseng with the power to prevent disease and treat sexual debility, sterility, fatigue, diabetes, anaemia, insomnia, depression and heart conditions.

The Russians became interested in ginseng during their involvement in Korea, where ginseng is widely used as a medicine. They took thousands of samples and cuttings of the root and sent them back to the U.S.S.R. for propagation. Soviet scientists certainly knew about ginseng because a variety, *Eleutherococus senticosus*, grows wild in Siberia. However, this is so valued by the local people that they secretly dug up the root and hoarded it so effectively that the authorities were prevented from ever getting a good supply to carry out research.

Ironically, owing to some interesting border smuggling, Siberian ginseng is now cultivated in the West.

The first analysis of ginseng at the Institute of Biologically Active Substances in Vladivostok described the root as having 'rare properties'.

Professor Brekhman then did the first research on ginseng. He devised a test in which mice were made to swim until they were exhausted. Selected mice were then given ginseng, and all the mice put back in the water. Those who had taken ginseng were able to go on swimming, whereas the others had to be fished out. If the mice were given ginseng regularly for a month, the extra stamina lasted for at least two months afterwards.

In another controlled experiment, scientists at the Institute gave ginseng to half the proofreaders of a newspaper to test their speed and accuracy. Those who had taken ginseng increased the amount they read by 12 per cent, and decreased the number of mistakes by 51 per cent.

At the Institute of Advanced Medical Training in Sofia, Professor Petkov carried out fifteen years of research into ginseng. He found that ginseng actually increased the efficiency of cerebral activity, and that brainwave patterns in both animal and human subjects increased in speed. In 1976 he wrote:

Ginseng stimulates the basic neural processes which constitute the functioning of the cerebral cortex, namely the excitation ... and inhibition ... which form the physiological basis of man's mental functioning as a whole.

The scientists at Vladivostok and Sofia came to the conclusion that ginseng could 'enhance the natural resistance and recuperative powers of the body and have both stimulant and sedative activities'.

The last phrase is particularly interesting. So many natural medicines can be both sedative and stimulant, showing that the combination of active constituents can act on the body in different ways at different times.

Professor Petkov commented:

Ginseng, in contrast to other stimulants, causes no disturbance in the equilibrium of the cerebral processes. This explains the absence of any pronounced sense of subjective excitement as is characteristic of all other stimulants ... and also why this stimulant does not interfere with the normal bodily functions.

After years of rigorous research, the Russians listed ginseng as a natural adaptogen, which they define as 'a substance which can help the body adapt to a broad spectrum of emotional and physical stresses and increase general resistance to disease'.

The value of such a medicine occurring naturally is beyond calculation.

In 1962 the Pharmacological Committee of the U.S.S.R. approved ginseng for clinical use and it has been prescribed by doctors ever since for quite an astonishing list of illnesses ranging from nerves to loss of virility.

Soviet astronauts are now given ginseng to increase their stamina and resistance whilst in orbit. Soviet athletes are given ginseng tablets and teas and the dosage is increased during the run-up to the Olympic Games.

In the West generally, scientists have remained cynical or baffled by ginseng. To a certain extent, this is because the man-shaped root still retains its ancient air of mystery. Many of its active constituents have yet to be identified and almost defy clinical analysis.

In the U.S.A., where American ginseng (*Panax quinquefolium*) has a long and honourable folk use as a medicine, its use as a drug was removed from the pharmacopoeia in 1960. There are some signs that scientific interest is being rekindled. One country doctor, in Alabama, was so intrigued by ginseng and its effects, particularly the American Indian uses of it, that he gave up his practice to devote his life to studying the enigmatic root.

The American *Pharmacognosy* (sixth edition) sums up the position fairly and neatly:

Scientists in Western countries have been unable to isolate physiologically active constituents from ginseng. Chinese and Soviet sources report a large number of physiologically active compounds, mostly glycosides which unfortunately have not been characterized structurally. These include: panaquilin, a glycoside said to stimulate endocrine secretions; panacin, a reported brain stimulant and cardiovascular tonic; panaxic acid, an 'aid' to heart and blood vessels; panacen, an analgetic and tranquilizer; ginsnenin, an anti-diabetic substance. The identity and physiological activity of these compounds require verification.

In West Germany a group of doctors found that patients with

high blood pressure made a small but significant improvement after taking ginseng.

At the University of Bonn, Dr Karzel carried out tests on ginseng's effect on sexual activity. He reported:

The occurrence of constituents with sex-like hormone-like activity in ginseng preparations thus seems to be proven . . . but questions concerning the ratios between male and female hormones remain to be solved.

This German finding certainly ties in with one Russian test at Kaschenko hospital, where six patients had to be taken off their course of ginseng due to an embarrassing increase in their sexual activities.

> **Constituents** <

Asiatic ginseng (*Panax ginseng*) contains several individual glycosides, some as yet unidentified, panax acid, saponins, other acids, essential oil, vitamin B, sugar, mucin, flavonoids, and starch.

American ginseng (*Panax quinque folium*) contains the glycoside panaquilin, panacin, saponins, and essential oils.

> **History** <

Ginseng has insignificant leaves on top of the ground but below the soil it possesses a most peculiar man-shaped root which has given rise to many legends. One Chinese story describes how the villagers of Shantan, in the Shensi province, were awakened each night by a terrible wailing. They took up torches and staves and tracked the sound to a nearby wood. There they dug up a huge root shaped exactly like a man with arms and legs, which shrieked as they pulled it up out of the ground. Even now, certain ceremonies are performed when ginseng roots are pulled up. The plant is addressed with these words: 'O ginseng, I need your powers, that is why I pull you up.' In the West, the mandrake, also shaped rather like a man, has had similar legends woven around it and was mentioned several times by Shakespeare in his plays. Men would blindfold themselves or tie the root to a dog before pulling it up.

The intriguing ginseng plant has never been cheap. There are several reasons contributing to this: it takes at least five years to develop fully and lives in mountainous areas or shady woods, which makes it difficult to find, so much so, that it is often called 'the root that hides from man'.

In China when supplies of ginseng were scarce, a rigorous class distinction was applied to would-be buyers. The Emperor got his ginseng first, then the court officials, aristocrats and so on. One Emperor paid the equivalent of £5,000 for a well-developed root.

The earliest Chinese book on the medicinal value of herbs was written by Emperor Shen-ung in about 3,000 B.C. He described ginseng as 'a tonic to the five viscera, quieting the animal spirits, strengthening the soul, allaying fear, expelling evil effluvia, brightening the eyes, opening the heart, benefiting the understanding, and if taken for some time it will invigorate the body and prolong life'.

In 1711 a Jesuit father, Jartoux, went to K'ang-hsi, and experienced at first hand the healing wisdom of the Chinese people. He sent a letter to the Royal Society in London describing 'a Tartarian plant, called ginseng'. With extraordinary intuition, Father Jartoux added: 'If it is to be found in any other country in the world, it may be particularly in Canada, where the forests and mountains . . . very much resemble those here.'

This account was read by another priest, Father Joseph Francis Lafitau, who was fascinated by these predictions. He wrote: 'After spending three months looking for the ginseng, by accident I found it. It was ripe, and the colour of the fruit attracted my attention. I pulled it up, and with joy, took it to an Indian I had engaged to help me hunt for it. She recognized it at once as one of the plants that the Indians used.'

As the value of ginseng became more widely known, American

ginseng was established as a near relative of the valuable Eastern root, sharing many of its virtues. On the principle that you can sell ice to Eskimos, enterprising American traders began exporting large quantities of ginseng to China and the East.

One ship sailed from Boston for China in 1773 with 55 tons of ginseng on board. Ships' captains used to offload their American ginseng and fill their holds to bulging point with teas, silks and spices for the return journey.

Ginseng is a fabled plant in Russia and there is a widespread belief that Rasputin used ginseng to achieve his amazing effects on the Czar's son. George St George wrote in *Russian Folk Medicine*:

It is generally believed that the infamous Rasputin's ability to stop the Czarevich's [Alexis] haemorrages, caused by haemophilia, was based on his use of some ginseng preparations, rather than on the power of his prayers. This is quite possible since Rasputin came from Siberia and, while in St Petersburg, had formed a close personal friendship with Dr Badmayer, the celebrated practitioner of Oriental medicine. Of course, this cannot be proved and must always remain a fascinating speculation.

> ## Folk Use <

In Eastern folk use, ginseng is quite simply the best natural medicine that money can possibly buy. First and foremost, it is widely valued as an aphrodisiac which can promote sexual virility well into old age.

In the Vedas, the old Indian scriptures, there is a hymn to ginseng describing it as 'the root which is dug from the earth and strengthens the nerves'. It goes on:

The strength of the horse, the mule, the ram, even the strength of the bull it bestows on him. This herb will make thee so full of lusty strength that thou shalt, when excited, exhale heat as a thing on fire.

In folk medicine, ginseng is strongly linked with maintaining youthful vigour and longevity. On a day to day basis, ginseng is used to keep the body in good health, create more energy and prevent disease. It is taken to fight tiredness, heart disease, painful periods, insomnia, diarrhoea, diabetes, indigestion, gout, rheumatism, coughs and colds – in short, a complete panacea.

A general tonic is made by infusing ginseng root with licorice root, mandarin orange rind and sweet basil. For flu, ginseng is infused with cassia bark, the roots of licorice, peony and ginger. A strengthening mixture taken during pregnancy and to ease childbirth is made by infusing ginseng root with betelnut, lovage, licorice and peony root and lemon rind.

On the other side of the world, the American Indians had discovered the value of their own ginseng. Many Indian tribes were quite friendly to the early settlers, showing them which native plants were good to eat. Ginseng, however, they kept secret and sacred until traders lured it from them with high prices.

The Alabama Indians drank ginseng juice to heal sores; the Houma drank the juice to control vomiting and ease the pain of rheumatism; the Penaobscots believed that ginseng increased fertility in women.

> Herbal Medicine <

Herbalists consider ginseng to be a fine natural rejuvenator and recommend it in all disorders of old age. Treatment consists of a three-month course of ginseng, three times a day, either in tablet form or ginseng tea made from a decoction of the shredded root. Half a teaspoon of shredded root is boiled in one cup of water for one minute, then left to stand for 15 minutes.

In America, the talented Shaker herbalists established the tradition of using ginseng as a tonic and a stimulant. They also dispensed ginseng elixirs for nervous debility, loss of appetite, weak stomach and asthma.

Ginseng is widely prescribed by herbalists for exhaustion, especially nervous exhaustion, and low blood pressure. It is strongly advised to be taken during times of stress. In all cases, ginseng tablets can be used if the root is hard to obtain.

> ## Culinary Use <

Ginseng is normally taken as tea, either ready to use as in tea bags or powders, or decocted from the root. Many people find it easier to take their ginseng in tablet or capsule form. All preparations use five- or six-year-old roots and this, no doubt, contributes to the high price.

There are several main categories of ginseng: Asiatic ginseng (*Panax ginseng*) which comes from China and Korea and is cultivated in Japan; American ginseng (*Panax quinquefolium*); Himalayan ginseng (*pseudoginseng*). Siberian ginseng is closely related but correctly called *Eleutherococus senticosus*.

Ginseng roots can be red or white, depending on the curing process. With American ginseng, six- to eight-year-old roots are lifted in the autumn and dried by artificial heat or in the sun. Asiatic red ginseng is produced by treatment with steam or hot water.

The Chinese Materia Medica lists the ginsengs in order of quality: first, the Manchurian white root, rarely seen outside China; second, the Chinese and Korean red and white roots; third, the Japanese cultivated plants; and finally, the American ginseng roots. Siberian ginseng is listed officially in the Russian pharmacopoeia.

> HONEY <

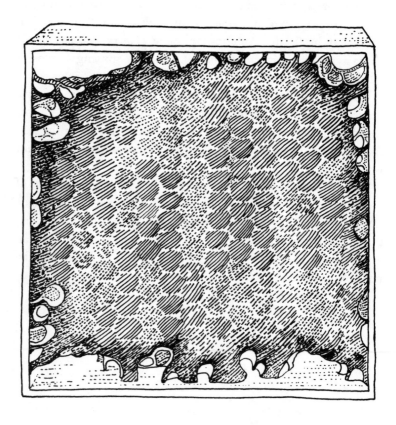

'My son, use thou honey for it is good,' said Solomon the wise in the Old Testament. Honey has held a special place in man's emotions ever since the Israelites were promised 'a land flowing with milk and honey'.

Emotions still run hotly on the 'goodness' of honey. On the one hand, health food enthusiasts believe that honey is a superfood for vitality and long life; on the other hand, orthodox medicine sees honey as a rich source of natural sugars.

To present a balanced argument one must say that honey is a highly concentrated source of sugars, and sugar whether natural or otherwise should never be taken to excess. Doctors now believe that too much sugar dangerously overloads the system and leads to obesity and illnesses such as diabetes.

After making that point, it is fair to say that honey is a very special food. It is a natural antiseptic with the proven power to kill germs. Honey combs and honey cappings can possess natural antibiotic qualities. The natural hormones in royal jelly are well publicized and much sought by middle-aged women who want to retain their youthful bloom.

Ordinary table honey contains a formidable combination of vitamins, sugar, minerals, acids, and enzymes.

Although honey has been used for over 10,000 years and subjected to close laboratory analysis for the past fifty years, there are several constituents which have not yet been identified.

The scientific approach to honey's wonder food reputation is that the balance of minerals and enzymes probably acts as a catalyst on bodily processes.

Honey is certainly more easily digested than white sugar. The bee has predigested the nectar, so the sugars are already converted into a readily available form. Other sugars need a complicated digestive process, but honey can go straight into the blood stream. This gives a powerful boost to energy much appreciated by athletes.

As well as being kind to the digestion, honey is also mildly laxative. It is especially suitable for small children and anyone recuperating from an illness. Research by Dr Schult and Dr Knott at the University of Chicago showed that babies tolerate and assimilate honey better than other sugars.

Honey has the advantage over sugars ... since it does not cause the blood sugar to rise to higher levels than can be easily cared for by the body.

The doctors noted also that infants fed on honey rarely have colic, since the rapid absorption prevents fermentation from taking place, and conclude: 'It is strange that honey has not enjoyed a wider use especially in the feeding of infants and children.'

Properly used, honey is excellent. The trouble is, many people think that if a small amount of something is good, a large amount must be even better. Homeopathy, with its minute doses, has disproved this notion. Real 'sweet tooth' cravings can gradually be curbed, and honey is generally preferable to white sugar.

Solomon was right. Honey *is* good. Use it as a soothing folk medicine when you need it, and, in moderation, as a flavour for daily food and drinks.

> **Constituents** <

Honey contains vitamins B1, B2, B3, B6 and folic acid, and it can contain large amounts of vitamin C. Naturally, this varies with the type of nectar. Very efficient filtering processes may remove some of the vitamins. In fact, honey is an excellent medium for vitamin stability.

The minerals in honey are iron, copper, sodium, potassium, manganese, calcium, magnesium and phosphorus. Natural sugars represent a major constituent, as do amino and other acids. Honey also contains several enzymes. Generally speaking, the darker the honey, the more minerals and vitamins present. Unfortunately, honey is often artificially darkened. The only way to be sure is to buy guaranteed honey from a specialist shop.

➤ History ◄

The prophet Mohammed is quoted as teaching: 'Honey is a remedy for every illness, and the Koran is a remedy for all illnesses of the mind. Therefore I recommend you to both remedies, the Koran and honey.' Mohammed referred to honey in many of his allegories. In one story a man went to the prophet and said his brother was ill with pains in his stomach. Mohammed told him to give his brother honey. Later the man returned and said his brother was no better. Mohammed said: 'Go back and give thy brother more honey for God speaks the truth; thy brother's body lies.' Given more honey as instructed, the man recovered.

In the Middle East honey has assumed an almost mystic quality over the centuries. In the Hindu marriage ceremony honey and curds are given to the groom when he enters the bride's home. Honey is part of the ritual, and as the groom kisses the bride he recites: 'Honey, this is honey, the speech of thy tongue is honey; in my mouth is the honey of the bee, in my teeth lives peace.'

When Pliny the Elder was travelling to collect material for his monumental work *Natural History*, he visited Africa, Britain, Spain and many Mediterranean countries. He came to the conclusion that honey promoted long life and vitality. Between the River Po and the Apennines he found a group of bee-keepers and recorded that 124 had passed the century age, the oldest being 135 years old. When he visited Britain, Pliny noted wryly that the inhabitants consumed vast quantities of honey, especially in the form of intoxicating mead. 'These islanders consume great quantities of honey brew,' he wrote.

The great folk authority on honey is Dr D. C. Jarvis, the Vermont country physician who made a life-long study of folk use in his native mountain state. His best-selling book, *Folk Medicine* (published by Pan Books, 1961) should really be credited with bringing this ancient subject back to common knowledge.

Dr Jarvis gives seven main reasons for using honey and not sugar:

1. It is non-irritating to the lining of the digestive tract.
2. It is easily and rapidly assimilated.
3. It quickly satisfies the demand for energy.
4. It enables athletes and others who spend energy heavily to recover rapidly from exertion.
5. It has a natural and gentle laxative effect.
6. It has a sedative value.
7. It is easier for the kidneys to process honey than all the other sugars.

Dr Jarvis noted that his Vermont patients instinctively treated arthritis, bedwetting, nervousness and sleeplessness with tablespoon doses of honey.

Observing his patients closely, Dr Jarvis found that honeycomb was even more effective than plain honey in some cases. The Vermont people chewed honeycomb as vigorously as a plug of chewing gum right throughout the hay fever season and whenever they had stuffy or blocked noses. Real hay-fever sufferers would start chewing honeycomb or honey cappings one month before the pollen count was started.

In their folk uses of honey the Vermont mountain people neatly encompass all the centuries-old traditions and remedies still valid in many countries of the world.

In France, liquid honey is mixed with olive oil or other agents to make an ointment for cuts, scars and minor burns. In Scandinavia honey and cod liver oil are used as a skin beautifying ointment. In China ginseng root and dried orange peel are chopped up and mixed with honey to make an effective vitalizer.

Every aspect of the bee's life and work has been studied by folk medicine. Pollen has a tremendous reputation as an energizer and is an ancient folk remedy for sexual impotence in men.

In primitive folk lore, royal jelly is believed to hold one of the secrets of eternal youth. It is especially associated with the prevention of wrinkled and sagging skin. In Papua and New Guinea tribes the women rub royal jelly and honey on their breasts to keep them firm and young. This practice is followed by tribeswomen in several other continents.

> Herbal Medicine <

Every branch of alternative medicine is united in recommending honey in preference to any other sweetening for general use. It is recommended as a strengthening dietary aid for anyone who is run down or edgy, irritable and nervy. For habitual constipation, a honey and apple cider vinegar drink is advised first thing in the morning on an empty stomach. The proportion is two tablespoons of honey to one tablespoon of cider vinegar; dilute with hot water.

Honey is often combined with other powerful natural medicines, such as onion, to treat bronchitis, flu and stuffy colds. Dilute honey is used as a gargle for ulcerated throats. A herbal gargle for sore throats is made with two tablespoons of honey, two tablespoons of dried or fresh sage, two tablespoons of cider vinegar and enough hot water to make the mixture fluid. Strain before use. Almond oil or clove oil can be added to this gargle, which also makes a most refreshing mouthwash.

> Culinary Use <

The composition of honey depends on flowers, the weather, the season and irresistible variations of nature. An extra flow of nectar from plants attracts bees at different times. In this way, with the help of a skilled bee-keeper, we get honey from an identified source, such as heather honey, clover honey, eucalyptus honey, or acacia blossom honey. It is well worth buying a good honey, because in some cheaper brands the bees are fed on a sugar solution placed just outside the hive. This short-cut method means that the complicated enzyme reaction does not take place.

Honey should always be kept covered in a dry place at room temperature. It is important to use a tight-fitting lid because honey is hygroscopic – which means that it attracts moisture. Honey tends to go darker and taste stronger with age. It can crystallize with very old age or if the temperature is too cool. To make it liquid again, put the honeypot in a pan of warm water and gently heat. When a good brand of honey is rather cloudy, this means that the pollens and other valuable nutrients have not been filtered out.

In cooking, honey can replace sugar in the majority of recipes. Use three-quarters the amount of honey and reduce any liquid by a fifth for each half cup of honey used.

Honey products are always available from specialist shops and are becoming increasingly popular in chain stores. These include:

Honeycomb: The hexagonal cells of wax that the bees make to support the honey.

Honey cappings: When the honey is ripe, the bee caps the cell with a layer of wax.

Propolis: The substance manufactured by bees to glue the hive together. Available in liquid and tablet form, and also as pleasant-tasting sweets.

Royal jelly: The jelly-like honey which the bees make to feed the young queen. A worker bee can be turned into a queen simply by eating this jelly, which is rich in natural hormones and enzymes.

Pollen: The pollen is collected, carefully screened of many allergic factors and made into tablets. Pollen tablets are valued by athletes in training.

Bee brood: When bees do not survive the winter, the larvae are marketed as a delicacy and can be fried, smoked or grilled.

Mead: Honey is fermented to make this traditional old English alcoholic drink.

❯ HORSERADISH ❮

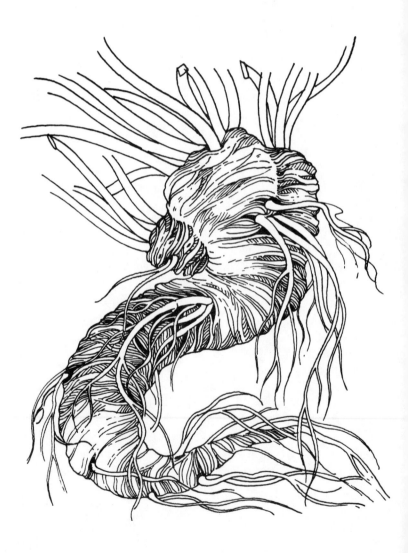

> Health <

If your eyes and nose stream when you eat horseradish sauce that is a fine indication that this herb is working on your system. Horseradish contains some dynamic ingredients including mustard oil, enzymes and a natural antibiotic agent. These active parts act dramatically on mucus throughout the body and cause the immediate running of nose and eyes from the moment a mouthful of horseradish is swallowed.

Of course, this attribute can be put to good use. Horseradish is wonderful for clearing stubborn catarrh and 'lifting' phlegm from the bronchial tubes. It is effective, too, against sinusitis, if used regularly.

Horseradish's combination of volatile oils and other active medicinal constituents is most unusual and exerts a splendid reviving effect on a weary or clogged-up system.

This herb is known to stimulate the metabolism, increase the stimulation of gastric juices, and also to have laxative and antiseptic as well as antibiotic powers.

In fact, a remarkable natural healer, but one which should never be taken in more than teaspoon-size amounts.

> Constituents <

Horseradish root contains essential oils with mustard oil, glycosides, enzymes, asparagin, vitamin B, iron and antibiotic substances.

> History <

Horseradish is native to Western Asia and South Eastern Europe. It has been cultivated in Central Europe since the twelfth century, first of all by the slaves who appreciated its pungent medicinal qualities. This herb is a classical botanic 'escape' story. Cultivated roots escaped to the wild, and being a rampant, galloping herb, horseradish now flourishes wild in many parts of the world.

The herbalist Gerard described horseradish growing in the

wild, confident that his readers were using it medicinally. What he strongly suspected, however, was that his fellow countrymen had no idea how to use horseradish as a vegetable. So he wrote:

The Horse Radish stamped with a little vinegar put thereto, is commonly used among the Germans for sauce to eate fish with and such like meates as we do mustarde.

Half a century later, horseradish was being used as a condiment as well as a natural drug. Parkinson described its use 'as a sauce with country people and strong labouring men in some countries of Germany', and adds, 'and in our owne land also, but, as I said, it is too strong for tender and gentle stomaches'.

> **Folk Use** <

Horseradish is one of the great 'spring cleansers' used traditionally in April or May to revitalize our systems after winter. A classic folk spring tonic is made from one teaspoon of shredded horseradish root, four large chopped stalks of celery, one teaspoon of dandelion root (optional). Place all the ingredients in a saucepan, cover with water, bring to the boil and simmer for about 20 minutes. In France they steep the same ingredients in brandy for a few days, and this preserves more of the active, volatile constituents. The mixture is then taken in teaspoon amounts four times a day for six days.

The antibiotic and germ-killing properties of horseradish have long been appreciated. In places like Siberia, where doctors are few and far between, the people make a medicine from horseradish, garlic and honey. It smells strong, but it works wonders.

In Russia, horseradish poultices and ointments are rubbed on the chest and legs to relieve congestion during bronchitis. These fiery applications also relieve rheumatism and arthritis, but they have to be carefully handled or they can cause the skin to blister. For external applications the root is always wrapped in muslin or cotton and the skin protected with a layer of olive oil.

Strangely enough, in view of horseradish's noted stimulant properties, there are no lovely risqué folk stories about its effect on sex life. Perhaps this is because it is neither possible nor desirable to eat more than minute amounts of this potent root.

> Herbal Medicine <

Horseradish is greatly valued for its expectorant qualities in herbal medicine, where it is used as a solvent for mucus in the bronchial tubes, nose and sinus. In fact, it is a specific remedy for sinus troubles. Half a teaspoon of freshly grated horseradish is taken in the morning and afternoon. The dose is taken at least half an hour before eating or drinking anything else. Sinus victims report that after horseradish medicine they feel a powerful sensation in the head, sometimes with sweating, often accompanied by spontaneous tears. Gradually these violent sensations decrease, and the sinus condition begins to improve.

The mucus-shifting qualities of horseradish are used by herbalists to treat persistent catarrh and bronchitis.

Horseradish's antibiotic and diuretic actions are also used in herbal medicine to treat bladder and kidney disorders. It is taken internally, in teaspoon amounts, to treat neuralgia and rheumatic complaints. Horseradish is also a herbal specific against jaundice and water retention.

Horseradish most definitely causes the gastric secretions to flow and therefore promotes digestion. In this way, it can act against indigestion, but it is not advised for those with delicate stomachs. For them, horseradish's powerful constituents should be taken in minute doses, or even more easily, as the French do, in alcoholic tinctures.

> Culinary Use <

The active ingredients of the root become inert when heated, so it is never worth adding to cooked dishes. In any case, the pungency is also lost, so little flavour is gained.

Luckily, fresh raw horseradish root is delicious freshly grated and made into sauces or relishes.

Old-fashioned horseradish relish has become a connoisseur's delight. Many good horseradish sauces are on the market now, but it is very easy to make yourself. Scrub the root well, dry and finely grate it; add finely grated turnip, spices, egg yolks, vinegar and enough soya flour to thicken nicely. Buzz in the blender or beat by hand to a sauce.

Horseradish is the main ingredient in *moutardes des allemandes*, where it combines with a mixture of vinegar, wine, cream, spice, mustard and seasoning which is excellent with sausages or salami.

Horseradish root can be grated and added sparingly to salad dressings and other sauces or made into sandwich spread. Notice that if other herbs are used at the same time, horseradish enhances the taste of the mixture.

Horseradish is an excellent condiment for those trying to follow a salt-free diet. It is also useful to anyone trying to get acquainted with grated raw food. Even in small quantities, it adds to the tastiness and helps one get accustomed to salt-free cooking.

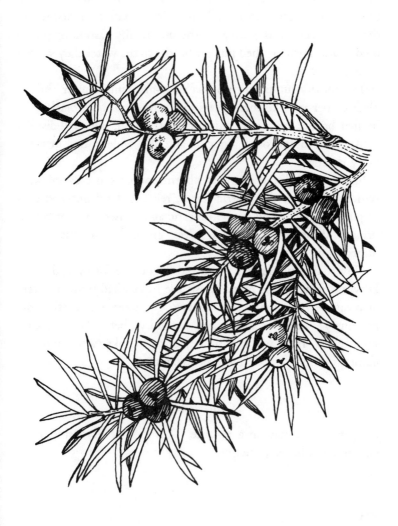

The juniper berry has a long convivial reputation in man's use of healing plants. Our word 'gin' is supposed to come from the French word for juniper – *genièvre*. Juniper berries are used to flavour gin and largely account for its unique taste.

Juniper is a natural antiseptic. Its strong germ-killing qualities were much appreciated in the past, especially during the terrible years of plague. Hygienic housewives burned spiky juniper branches and berries in their hearths in the safe knowledge that the sweet scent was purifying the air. Really fastidious people used to add a few crushed juniper berries to the water they washed their clothes in.

The thorny juniper shrub is a slow-growing conifer and the seeds or berries take three years to ripen to full blue-black. Ripe juniper berries are a rich source of volatile oil, which is distilled to flavour gin and other liqueurs and also widely used in veterinary practice.

Juniper oil is listed in many pharmacopoeias as a carminative which stimulates the gastric juices, relieves flatulence and eases griping pains. The oil is also diuretic and is used to treat certain urinary disorders, but it is never given for serious kidney disorders or during pregnancy.

Nowadays, juniper is a neglected flavouring for everyday use. Previous generations made lavish use of crushed juniper berries in meat stews or marinades for two good reasons: firstly, they genuinely liked the taste; and secondly, before refrigeration slightly 'off' meat was commonplace and cooks valued juniper's natural germicide action as a protection.

> **Constituents** <

Juniper berries contain a volatile oil, a flavone glycoside, resin, tannin and a bitter principle.

> History <

The juniper tree is revered in Catholic countries because of the tradition that when the Virgin Mary and the infant Christ were fleeing from Herod, they took refuge behind a juniper tree. Elijah was also protected from the persecution of Ahab by the juniper, and it has become a symbol of protection. 'Swete is the juniper but sharp his bough.'

According to Pliny, Hannibal commanded that the beams of the temple to Diana should be built of juniper for its long lasting and pure qualities.

> Folk Use <

Although the juniper tree grows naturally in Europe, North America, and Asia, it is the Europeans who have made most recorded use of the medicinal berry. The Dutch put the berries into gin while the rest of the Continent drank them in less pleasant-tasting teas and infusions as a prevention against the plague.

In the Mediterranean countries, sprays of juniper were hung on the door to keep away snakes and rodents. The branches were burned in the streets and all public places during epidemics and cholera. Hippocrates recorded that Athens was saved from the plague in this way.

In England, Gerard considered juniper 'a most admirable Counter-poyson' and a great 'resister of the Pestilance'.

During an outbreak of smallpox in Paris late last century, the time-honoured burning of juniper branches and berries was used to disinfect hospital wards.

Chewing juniper berries is a standard folk remedy for anyone who is in contact with sickness or who needs protection against fevers in tropical countries. The berries are also chewed or infused into a tea to treat bronchial catarrh, sluggishness and lack of appetite.

Juniper tea or wine is a classic treatment for really bad rheumatism. While juniper medicine is being taken, juniper ointment or liniment is also rubbed on the skin externally to relieve the rheumatic pains. Juniper wine is made by macerating or steeping 100 grams of berries in one litre of white wine for about five days in a warm place. The mixture is taken at about 15 or 20 drops a day, often on a lump of sugar. The liniment is made by macerating 100 grams of juniper berries in half a litre of olive oil for about 15 days. The liniment is rubbed onto the affected rheumatic joints and is also good for lumbago, sciatica and muscular pains in general.

Early colonists in the New World noted that the Indian braves washed their wounds immediately with juniper infusions. This Indian wisdom was shared by Europeans in the old world. With half a teaspoon of juniper berries to a cup of boiling water they made a fine natural germicide.

> Herbal Medicine <

Abbé Kneipp, the redoubtable German herbalist, felt quite passionately about the benefits of juniper.

I cannot understand the father or mother who, whilst carefully seasoning the family's meat and choucroute with salt and juniper, and meticulously filling their homes with the fragrance of juniper, will let the body, which is the dwelling place of the soul, wallow in filth and dust. This dwelling place too, from time to time during the year, needs fumigating and vaporizing with juniper: this cleanses the body and soothes the respiratory apparatus.

The Abbé's purifying treatment is still practised in Germany today. It consists of eating progressive amounts of berries, starting with four on the first day and increasing by one until fifteen are taken, then reducing again by one a day until the original amount of four is reached, a treatment lasting twenty-three days.

Internationally, herbalists use juniper to treat rheumatism, and a course of juniper tea is highly recommended for those who suffer chronically from this complaint. Under this system, juniper tea is taken twice a year in the spring and autumn. Pour one cup of boiling water over one teaspoon of well-crushed juniper berries; cover and let stand for 20 minutes. Strain and take one cup in the morning and one in the evening for four to six weeks in spring and autumn.

For cystitis, a cup of boiling water poured over one tablespoon of crushed berries is taken morning and evening for about one week or ten days.

Juniper berries are chewed for their antiseptic qualities during some stomach infections. In fact, European herbalists advise anyone predisposed to kidney stones to cultivate the old habit of chewing a few juniper berries regularly.

> **Culinary Use** <

Juniper is used traditionally to cure smoked meat, and this distinctive flavour can easily be achieved at home by adding a few berries to the charcoal fire when barbecuing meat. Another modern idea is to grind the juniper berries in a pepper pot or with pestle and mortar and sprinkle on meat or chops ready for the grill.

Juniper has fallen sadly out of use as a flavouring in England and America but the European tradition is still as strong as ever.

In Germany, juniper berries are added to sauerkraut and used as a spice for roast meat and sauces. French cooks use them for *choucroute*, salt meat and fish, marinades and *court bouillons*. Scandinavian countries make the berries into a *rob* which is good with cold meat. (A *rob* is the juice of a fruit or berry thickened by heat and preserved with honey.)

Besides its well-known addition to gin, juniper is used to flavour aquavit and some Scandinavian beers. In France, wine (*vin de genièvre*) is made from juniper berries with the occasional addition of absinthe.

The old imaginative uses of juniper as a condiment can easily be revived. Add a few berries to a ham when it is boiling, or put several crushed berries into any slow cooking beef dish to transform the flavour into something quite unusual.

When buying juniper berries, bear in mind that those from hot countries are stronger and can contain up to six times as much volatile oil as those from colder countries.

> LETTUCE <

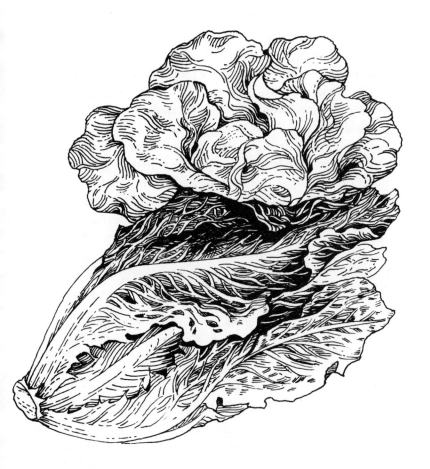

Think of salads, and a vision of the familiar green lettuce appears, either deliciously crisp and crunchy or sadly limp, resting under slices of tomatoes and cucumbers. What is to us a standard salad green vegetable was used by our ancestors with enormous respect as a natural tranquillizer and sedative.

Wild lettuce (*Lactuca virosa*) is narcotic, and all lettuce possesses some of the narcotic juices. Not enough to make anyone drugged or addicted, of course, but enough to justify its ancient reputation as a tranquillizer.

The scientific approach is based on the fact that lettuce, especially the stem, contains a white, milky latex which flows freely from the plant when it is wounded. This substance, known as lettuce-opium or lactucarium, is dried and used medically in pastels or lozenges as a sedative for irritating or hacking coughs. It is also used to treat bronchitis and asthma. Wild varieties of lettuce are specially grown for the chemical industry, which extracts the milky latex from them.

In France, *eau de laitue* is distilled from lettuce and prescribed as a mild sedative. The time-honoured lettuce teas and soups are another method of concentrating lettuces' powers. These home-made remedies are effective in their calming action and good for over-excited minds and sleeplessness.

Beatrix Potter, in *The Tale of the Flopsy Bunnies*, comments:

It is said that the effect of eating too much lettuce is 'soporific'.
I have never felt sleepy after eating lettuces; but then *I* am not a rabbit. They certainly had a very soporific effect upon the Flopsy Bunnies!

> **Constituents** <

Garden lettuce is rich in minerals and vitamins. It contains potassium, iron, copper, cobalt, zinc, calcium and the vitamins A, B and C with good amounts of vitamin E. Several alkaloids are present, and a small amount of lactucarium.

> History <

Lettuce was a medicinal plant of the Ancient Egyptians and Chinese. It features in the Passover ritual of the Hebrews along with Paschal Lamb. The Father of Medicine, Hippocrates, prescribed lettuce as a sedative. Illustrious Romans and commoners alike considered it a magnificent health food.

The Emperor Augustus believed the plant had cured him of a dangerous illness, so he built an altar to the honour of lettuce. Galen, too, thought that lettuce had saved his life and, what was more, brought him restful sleep. In Roman times lettuce was usually served at the end of the meal as a tribute to its sedative and calming properties. The Emperor Domitian insisted on having his lettuce first, causing the poet Martial to write: 'How comes it that this food which our ancestors ate only as a dessert is now the first that is put before us?'

After his abdication, the Emperor Diocletian turned a fine philosophical phrase when he was urged by a friend to return to power. He said: 'My friend, if you could see what fine lettuces I am growing, you would not urge me so hard to take up that burden again.'

> Folk Use <

The expressed juice of lettuce is one of the oldest soporifics. The juices and milky latex were used in folk lore very much as modern medicine uses them today. Lettuce leaves and stems were wounded and the droplets carefully dried on plates. The resulting powder (which we now know as lactucarium) was bound into white cakes and given to patients before and after surgical operations, together with poppy seed.

While lettuce is a treasured folk tranquillizer and aid for sleeplessness, it also has a sly reputation for quelling sexual ardour.

The Pythagoreans called it 'the plant of the Eunuch' and Dioscorides recommended the juice to control lust. Culpeper said: 'The juice of lettuce mixed with oil of roses, applied to the forehead and temples procures sleep and easeth the head-ache.' He then goes on to say: 'It abateth bodily lust.'

In the Middle Ages, knights departing for the Crusades locked their wives in chastity belts and bade them drink lettuce tea to 'quench the fires of lechery'.

This unwarranted reputation is no doubt due to the sedative, soporific effect that lettuce remedies can have, and should be tempered by the knowledge that relaxation can be good for sexual vigour too.

By one of the interesting ironies thrown up by folk medicine from time to time, lettuce juice is a remedy for men losing their hair. Tradition also has it that bald men are more virile!

For sleeplessness, a classic folk remedy is lettuce tea. A large lettuce is stripped, plucked into small pieces, covered with boiling water and simmered for about 20 minutes. The stem is cut gently with a knife and added to the tea for about five minutes of slow simmering. A potent folk tea against sleepless-ness is made by combining poppy seed, lettuce leaves and stem, and chamomile flower.

The French style is to combine the medicinal virtues with *haute cuisine* and braise several lettuces with bone-marrow. Not less than three lettuces should be used to treat insomnia.

> **Herbal Medicine** <

Herbalists use the milky juice from the fresh, wild or prickly lettuce to treat gout, asthma, jaundice and spasmodic coughing. The juice is sometimes made into pills or syrups to relieve coughs and insomnia. Garden lettuce juice is also used in medi-cines for certain nervous disorders, coughs and menstrual pain.

The lettuce seeds are also used in herbal medicine. Culpeper thought that seed infusions were good for 'over-heated urine'.

European herbalists use *eau de laitue* and other lettuce remedies to treat sleeplessness, especially when it is accompanied by over-excitability or sexual tension.

> **Culinary Use** <

Bear in mind that lettuce stems are rich in the medicinal juice, and treat 'run-to-seed' lettuces as a boon, rather than a nuisance. In French cooking, lettuce stalks are trimmed and cooked like asparagus. In British cooking the thicker lettuce stalks are made into a candied preserve, very like root ginger. The stalks are stripped of the tougher outer skin and well chopped.

A syrup is made from sugar (450 grams of sugar to each 450 grams of stem) and a knob of ginger root, poured on to the stems and brought to the boil. Remove from the heat and leave until next day. Then drain off the syrup, boil it up again and pour over the stems. Keep on doing this until the syrup is really thick and the stems have a clear, crystal look. The stems are bottled in jars with a pinch of citric acid to improve the keeping quality. This makes a cheap and impressive preserve, very like Chinese ginger.

There are two main types of lettuce: cabbage lettuce with large heads and round leaves, and cos lettuces with tall, oblong leaves and a generally sweeter flavour. Some lettuces, such as the American or 'Iceberg', are developed for their big hearts which are ideal in salads.

Lettuce's mineral and vitamin value are highest when we eat it fresh and raw in our familiar salads. The dark green outside leaves have as much as thirty times more value than the inner paler ones, so don't throw them away. Make outer or wilted leaves into soup with spring onions and a dash of cider vinegar. Braised whole lettuces can be a delicious hot vegetable, especially when cooked in chicken stock.

There is a time-honoured belief that the juices of lettuce bleed and go brown if it is cut with a knife. This is the reason why people pluck the leaves into pieces with their fingers.

> MUSTARD <

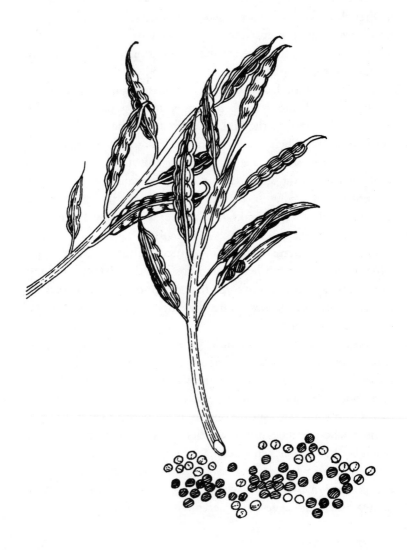

> Health <

The old saying 'as keen as mustard' describes the biting action of this spice to a nicety. Black mustard, like white mustard, is widely used as a condiment and also appreciated for its medicinal powers. Black mustard is used more medically because it produces a more powerful volatile oil.

Black mustard's strength is to increase the blood supply and to stimulate the skin locally. Mustard plasters are listed in many pharmacopoeias and are used in bronchitis and pleurisy. The warming and drawing effect of the plaster is also valuable in arthritis, sciatica and rheumatism.

Mustard, both black and white, stimulates the lining of the alimentary tract and increases the peristaltic action of the stomach. So it is deservedly known as a natural aid to digestion, and one that can counter the effects of fatty foods.

In larger doses, mustard is an emetic, a handy first aid in cases of accidental poisoning.

> Constituents <

Black mustard seed contains the enzyme myrosin, which produces a volatile mustard oil, sinigrin, proteins and mucilage.

White mustard seed contains myrosin and sinalbin, which produces a much less volatile oil than black mustard.

> History <

In Biblical times black mustard was very common in Palestine, and it occurs in one of the most vivid parables of Jesus:

'And he said, "With what can we compare the kingdom of God, or what parable shall we use for it? It is like a grain of mustard seed, which, when sown upon the ground, is the smallest of all the seeds on earth; yet when it is sown it grows up and becomes the greatest of all shrubs, and puts forth large branches, so that the birds of the air can make nests in its shade." '

This is a graphic reference to the tiny mustard seed which can grow rapidly into a tree three metres high in warm climates.

The Romans started the practice of mixing the sweet must of old wine with crushed seeds to make *mustum ardens* (hot must), hence the name mustard.

Black mustard was mentioned by Diocletian (300 A.D.), and both Theophrastus and Pliny mention its use as a medicine.

In the Middle Ages the monks throughout Europe grew mustard in monastery gardens for medicine and to preserve food. They found that the active ingredients in mustard inhibited bacteria and stopped food going off.

Throughout the ages mustard has been immensely popular in France, occasionally reaching heights of passion. When the Duke of Burgundy gave a feast in 1336, his almoner recorded that the guests ate seventy gallons of mixed mustard. Philippe the Bold was so delighted with the mustard made in Dijon that he granted the town its own armorial bearings in 1382.

In the eighteenth century a Mrs Clements of Durham invented the modern method of dressing mustard powder and earned herself a fortune.

> **Folk Use** <

Mustard's fiery power to stimulate and increase circulation of the skin was methodically used by the ancient Greeks for paralysed limbs. They massaged the joints with wine in the morning, olive oil in the evening, and throughout the day applied mustard poultices.

These poultices are a time-honoured way of treating acute local pains, such as rheumatism, arthritis, sciatica, lumbago and bronchitis. In England, mustard poultices were applied to the feet to improve circulation. Poultices are simply made by mixing mustard powder and cold water to a paste-like consistency and heating over a pan of boiling water then wrapping in cotton. A poultice should *never* be applied directly to the skin since it can produce painful blisters. It should also be covered with a layer of lint.

Hot mustard foot baths, so beloved by our Victorian ancestors, are still valued for their effective use in chills and colds. If you have been out in cold weather and are soaking and shivery, a hot mustard foot bath can prevent a cold or chill. They are especially valuable when a cold or 'fluey' feeling is made worse by wet feet. Mix a tablespoon of mustard into a paste and add it to a deep bowl of hot water. Bathe the feet for five or ten minutes.

Folk medicine also uses mustard powder added to baths for poor circulation and nervous tension, but this is not to be recommended for those with skin complaints.

In Siberia, workers swear by mustard powder sprinkled inside their socks each morning to keep colds at bay during the long harsh winter.

> **Herbal Medicine** <

European herbalists make a drink of bruised black mustard seeds to loosen mucus in respiratory infections and to stimulate circulation. The decoction is strained and taken in teaspoon doses for short periods.

The liquid also makes a mild gargle which quickly clears phlegm from the throat and sweetens bad breath.

Mustard is held to be a fine deodorizer; problem feet or armpits often respond to bathing with a mild mustard solution. (Never when there are any pimples or cuts on the skin.)

Mustard poultices are still used herbally, applied directly to the acute pain in lumbago and rheumatism, muscular aches, and to relieve congestion in bronchitis and pneumonia.

Eastern medicine uses hot mustard foot baths after reflexology or massage. Alternate hot and cold foot baths are valued as a stimulant to the system. Chinese doctors, in particular, believe that if the feet are aching and tired the whole body feels worn out. A Chinese instant reviver is to sit with the feet in a hot, stimulating bath, and an iced herbal compress on the back of the neck and over the eyes.

> ### > Culinary Use <

Black mustard is stronger and more pungent than white, so the two are often blended for the roundest flavour. French mustards are made from a mixture of white and black powdered mustard seed, often with herbs added. Dijon mustard is made with verjuice (unripened grape juice) whereas Bordeaux mustard uses ripe grape juice.

Dijon mustard has a fine, clean taste and is preferred in French sauces unless the recipe states otherwise.

German mustard is flavoured with herbs and spices. Its sweet-sour flavour goes well with sausages and cold meat.

In America, a thick, mild mustard has been evolved as the perfect accompaniment to hot dogs and hamburgers. Which only goes to show that each mustard, matched with care, can really enhance a meal.

Continental and American mustards come as ready-to-use pastes. In Britain the popular form is mustard powder, which has to be mixed by the cook. The important thing to remember is that the enzyme which produces the distinctive 'mustard oil' only starts action on contact with cold water. This is why powder should be stirred and left awhile before it becomes real mustard, and never poured straight into hot dishes as some recipes recommend.

The small leaves of mustard and cress which add zest to our salads are actually the seedlings of the plant, a few days old.

Many people, especially in Europe, enjoy the piquant taste of the white mustard leaves. (It is, after all, a member of the cabbage family.) The Romans loved them raw in salads but could never get the recalcitrant Britons to eat the leaves. Another milder variety (*Brassica juncea*) is grown in the Southern United States, where 'mustard greens' are standard vegetables.

Whole white seeds can be added to red or green cabbage while it is cooking. The seeds add flavour to pickles, chutneys and relishes. As a condiment, mustard has an affinity with meat, especially beef, and is a traditional ingredient of Welsh rarebit and toasted cheese. It is added by many expert cooks to their mayonnaises and salad dressings for an unusual flavour.

> OATS <

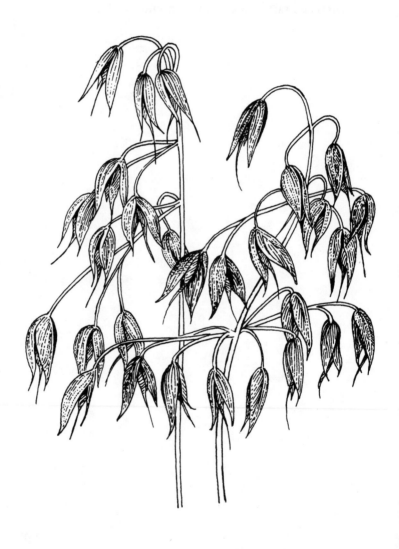

Oatmeal porridge, the traditional dish of Scotland, has a fine double-edged reputation. On the one hand, it is acknowledged as an easily digestible, nourishing dish, ideal during convalescence; on the other hand, it was the staple diet of the Scottish clans, and built brawny Highlanders and fiery warriors.

This is not Scots fantasy. From the thirteenth century, oats were a vital staple in the diet of the rural poor in Scotland. Frank Buckland, medical adviser to the British Army in the mid nineteenth century, wrote a report on the physical conditions of the recruits. The Scots soldiers he examined had lived mainly on oatmeal, milk and vegetable broths. Dr Buckland described their fine physique and compared them to the weedy Southerners. The Scots were taller and hardier.

In Switzerland last century Dr Bircher-Benner chose oats as the most digestible and soothing cereal, an ideal base for his now world-famous health food, muesli.

The medicinal uses of oats are divided between the grain and the stalks or straw of the plant. Our forebears noticed that horses eating oats in the field became excitable and frisky. Modern pharmacists have identified an alkaloid in the outer husks of the oat which acts on the central nervous system. The stalks or straw are known to stimulate skin metabolism and strengthen connective tissues. Homeopaths and herbalists make good use of these qualities.

The longstanding anti-depressant reputation of the oat grain prompted its use in orthodox medical experiments in Canada, Britain and Australia, with volunteers who were trying to overcome dependence on tobacco, opium or morphine. No definite conclusion could be drawn. However, in 1975, an experiment with rats in Britain showed that an alcoholic tincture of oats reduced physical dependence on morphine.

The de-husked oat is ground or rolled into oatmeal, and that is how most of us eat it. Oatmeal has its own medicinal qualities.

It is nutritious and soothing, rich in minerals, including calcium, magnesium and potassium, and a good source of B vitamins, particularly inositol which is needed for good eyesight, smooth skin and thick hair. Scots sailors and crofters prided themselves on their keen eyesight and healthy hair.

In everyday use, oatmeal is a proven softener and conditioner for the skin and has been known to heal inflamed patches of eczema. It is popular commercially in soaps, face cleansers and many other beauty aids.

For the best effect, use super-fatted colloidal oatmeal for beauty because it leaves the skin silky smooth, soft and clean. Make the oatmeal into face masks by simply mixing it to a stiff paste with milk or elderflower water, or throw a handful into the bath when the hot tap is running.

> **Constituents** <

Oatmeal contains B vitamins, especially inositol, flavone, the alkaloid trigonelline, saponins, fibre with moderate amounts of iron, potassium and linoleic acid. The stalk or straw is rich in silicic acid, saponins, mucins, vitamin A and calcium.

> **History** <

Although oats are known to have developed in about 2,500 B.C., they were regarded merely as a weed until the expanding Roman Empire needed more grain. The conquering legions carried oat seeds to Britain and found them well suited to the cool, wet climate. Oats gradually became an important staple in the diet of the rural poor, most notably in Northern England and Scotland.

Samuel Johnson is scathing about this Scottish staple food. In his dictionary (first edition 1755) he wrote: 'Oats – a grain, which, in England, is generally given to horses, but in Scotland, supports the people.'

A sea captain took oats with him to the New World in 1602 and planted them on the Elizabeth Isles off the coast of Massachusetts. The oat plant flourished on the coast and became popular in the Southern states. The colonists found that oatmeal porridge was a nourishing and sustaining food in hard times.

> Folk Use <

The fact that poor people in some rural areas *had* to eat porridge and gruel merely to keep from starvation makes their high reputation in folk medicine worth a second glance. Such familiarity made oats' special effects obvious.

Traditionally, oatmeal is regarded as a strengthening food with easily absorbed minerals, which builds good bones and muscles. Romany mothers give their growing children oatmeal jelly, and take it themselves when they are pregnant. Oatmeal is known to be kind to the digestion, and is standard folk food in illness or for anyone who is 'run down'.

Abbé Kneipp wrote in France during the nineteenth century: 'I often regret that the sick, whose blood needs purifying and fortifying, are given all kinds of beverage to drink but never a decoction of oats.' The Abbé listed the virtues of oats as 'easily digestible', 'cooling for over-heated blood', and 'an excellent restorative for convalescents exhausted by serious illness'.

The oat drink he recommended is easily made by cooking one cup of oat flakes in six cups of water until the liquid is reduced by half. Strain and drink. This beverage is diuretic and acts on the bladder and kidneys.

Oatmeal is esteemed, too, as a nerve strengthener, one of the finest folk remedies for calming irritable people who cannot sleep. In Wales, a bedtime drink called *stokos* is made with fine oatmeal and milk. Many traditional drinks are made with oatmeal, including one with ale called caudle. The soothing qualities of the oat have long been valued and used in gruels and drinks for sore stomachs and indigestion (not dyspepsia). Oatmeal is used in cases of diarrhoea; roasted oats are used as a laxative coffee where constipation is accompanied by haemorrhoids.

If the soothing properties of the oat were well observed, so were the excitant effects of the rest of the plant. Not knowing anything about alkaloids in the pericarp, country people boiled up the whole lot – straw, whiskers and all. The resulting drink enjoyed a wide reputation as a stimulant, especially to the sex glands. Oatmeal is still widely used as a skin conditioner, a beauty aid and a cleansing rub. It is particularly valuable for problem skins. A traditional Irish skin lotion is made by half filling a bottle with oatmeal and topping it up with boiled water. The bottle is turned upside down and the mixture is shaken regularly over 24 hours. The strained water is used as a lotion and considered excellent for cleansing the pores. In Ireland too, buttermilk and oatmeal are mixed into a face pack which conditions and whitens the skin.

> Herbal Medicine <

Medical herbalists often advise patients with colitis, ulcers or inflamed stomach conditions to start the day with finely ground oatmeal porridge. They also prescribe medicine made from the outer grain and stalk of the oat as a tonic and nerve restorative.

Eczema, dermatitis and other skin troubles, too, respond to prescribed oat herbal medicines. Anyone who does not have easy access to a registered herbalist might try the Irish skin lotion described above in *Folk Use*.

Some naturopaths value a tincture of black oats as a remedy against cyclic depression and the resulting loss of vitality.

> Homeopathic Medicine <

Homeopathic chemists use various parts of the oat plant to make Avena Sativa, the homeopathic remedy. This oat medicine is a favourite remedy for insomnia, especially that associated with nervous or general fatigue. This remedy is used when sleeplessness brings lack of general muscle tone and day-long fatigue and debility. It is also prescribed for lack of appetite following a prolonged illness, or when general run-down feelings and fatigue follow a feverish ailment.

> ## > Culinary Use <

Groats are oat grains with the outer husk removed. The groat skin is milled off to make the oat or oatmeal which we are most familiar with. Oats can be left coarse or rolled into smaller, softer pieces which are quicker to cook. For muesli bases, the oatflakes are preferred large but not coarse.

While most of us think of oatmeal in terms of porridge or muesli, it can be a very versatile food. In Ireland, roasted oatmeal is made into vegetarian sausages. The English county of Lincolnshire perfected unleavened oatmeal bread, an English equivalent of pitta bread. It was split and stuffed with bacon for hungry labourers' lunch packs. In the U.S.A., oatmeal is an ingredient of Boston brown bread, cookies, muffins, parkin, blintzes, and kasha.

In France, crushed groats are made into soup (*potage a l'avoine au naturel*). The Scots still excel in their imaginative use of oats, and Scottish recipes may be found for: oatcake, gruel, bannocks, puddings, flummery, dumplings, sowans, brose, boose, hodgils and skerlie.

The Scots prefer coarse oatmeal for their porridge, and say that the secret of thick non-lumpy porridge is to bring the water to a rolling boil, add a pinch of salt, and let the oats trickle gradually into the water from a clenched fist.

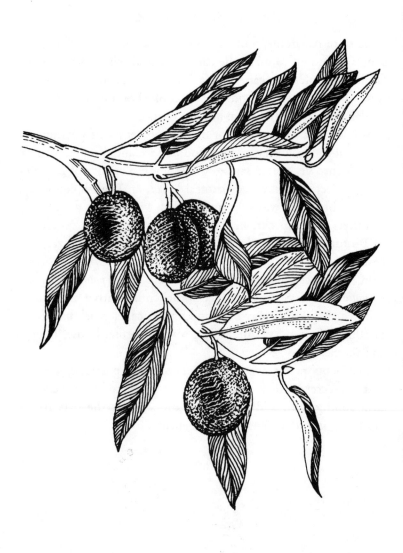

The olive tree, symbol of peace and prosperity, is also the source of an important natural medicine. Olive oil is recognized in the British, U.S. and many other pharmacopoeias as soothing, nutrient, and laxative.

Olive oil is recognized as a safe, effective laxative. Holiday visitors to Greece, Italy or other Mediterranean lands where olive oil is widely used in cooking can vouch for its efficacy in what used to be coyly called inner cleanliness. If you are not used to olive oil, even a visit to a Continental restaurant can have noticeable results.

For this reason, if you are a newcomer to olive oil, start taking it in small amounts, half a teaspoon to begin with and gradually work up. After all, several pharmacopoeias recommend olive oil as a purgative in doses from 15 to 60ml (or just over one to four tablespoons). French herbalists happily recommend olive oil in wine glass amounts medicinally, safe in the knowledge that their patients have been using it since birth.

Olive oil has an entirely soothing effect, making it useful in indigestion. Medically, the emollient qualities are used on the skin to soothe inflamed surfaces and soften crusts in eczema and psoriasis.

Regularly used, olive oil can help keep skin healthy and young. It is one of the most easily absorbed of oils and leaves the skin smooth and springy. All in all, a wonderful beauty aid.

Yet this is another good food shunned by overweight people on diets, and a superficial glance shows that olive oil calories are about 125 per tablespoon. American research has shown that cutting oil or fats completely out of the diet often has the opposite effect to that intended, and can cause fluid retention or swelling. Some doctors also believe that complete oil or fat-free diets have a bad effect on the production of female hormones. Adelle Davis put forward the theory that only when fat enters the intestines does the gall bladder empty itself vigorously. Add to this olive oil's known stimulating action on the secretion of bile, and you have a dieting friend, not a foe.

It is significant that the International Slimming Organization, Weight Watchers, have made a major policy change to their standard programme. Dieters are now recommended to take up to two tablespoons of fresh, uncooked vegetable oil each day.

When olive oil is used for health, it is obviously worth buying the purest quality. An expert Continental cook will give the same care to choosing the oil that connoisseurs give to their wine. It should be said that in non-olive-producing countries, finding a good, pure oil is like tiptoeing through a minefield. Undoubtedly, the finest quality is virgin oil with its characteristic light greenish colour. The difficulty comes because manufacturers do not relate olive oil grades to the actual production process.

General modern factory practice is to extract the oil from the de-stoned fruit by hydraulic pressure. Virgin oil comes from very gentle pressure on the peeled pulp; first and second grade oil is produced by increasing pressure on the same pulp, now crushed. For third or industrial grade oil the fruit pulp is washed with hot water and crushed, or extracted with carbon disulphide. The worst oil, ungraded, or called Turkey Red Oil (in the U.S.A.) comes from windfall olives which have been allowed to ferment.

Olive oil can go rancid, too, if it is stored incorrectly in shops. Many people owe their dislike of olive oil to either rancidity or poor quality. Then again, oil from different countries has different textures. Italian is fruitier than French for instance, and may suit some people better. The residents of Provence in France and Lucca in Italy each claim to produce the best olive oil in the world. California could now rival that claim. Generally, avoid oil which is the product of more than one country. Experiment with the different olive oils and find one that suits you. Use a good retailer, preferably one who knows his importers. Very often small ethnic shops, such as Greek or Italian, sell very fine olive oil, simply because their customers demand it.

> Constituents <

The drupe or fruit of the olive is rich in oleic acid with linoleic acid, arachidic acid, traces of lecithin, enzymes, and a bitter principle. Both green and black olives contain calcium, iron, sodium, potassium, vitamin A and fibre. Pickled green olives contain about four times as much sodium as ripe olives, and about four times as much vitamin A. The fibre content is lost in the oil-making process.

> History <

Noah knew when the great flood was over because the dove flew back to the ark with an olive branch in his beak. In the ancient world the olive tree was both a symbol of purity and peace and an emblem of prosperity. Moses exempted from military service men skilled in olive culture. The olive is thought to be native to Palestine, but the Ancient Greeks claimed it as their own. Herodotus wrote: 'At a time not long past there was not an olive tree in the world except those at Athens.' In Greek mythology the goddess Hera bathed in perfumed olive oil to tempt Zeus, and Achilles washed his horses' manes with it. Like the Hebrews, the Greeks honoured the olive tree as a symbol of purity and were strict about those who tended it. At one stage, only chaste men and virgins were allowed to tend the olives. The Romans, too, venerated the olive tree and it gradually became the universal symbol of peace. For centuries warring armies 'extended the olive branch' to call a ceasefire. Today it is an emblem on the United Nations flag and an olive branch is the torch which carries the sacred Olympic flame to each Olympic games.

> Folk Use <

Olive oil is one of the great folk medicines of the Mediterranean, and has always been valued for beneficial effects inside the body and beautifying effects on skin and hair.

As a medicine, olive oil is a traditional European aid during liver troubles. Virgin olive oil has a reputation as an anti-alcohol agent and a friendly aid to troubled livers. In Europe a popular cure for irritated livers is a tablespoon of olive oil each morning, often with a few drops of lemon juice to help it down. Folk medicine believes that the oil is better digested and absorbed with a few drops of lemon juice.

A large spoonful of olive oil before parties is an old and sound English folk prevention against drunkenness and hangovers. Sir Hugh Platt advised in his *Jewell House of Art and Nature* in 1594: 'Drinke first a good large Draught of Sallet oyle [olive oil], for that will float upon the Wine which you shall drinke, and suppresse the spirits from ascending into the braine.' The scientific theory behind this advice is that any fat in the stomach delays absorption of alcohol. When alcohol passes more slowly into the blood it does not have the same effect on the nervous system.

Folk medicine uses olive oil as a remedy whenever soothing action is needed, such as in inflammation or ulceration of the stomach, colic and bile stones. The gentle laxative action is used as a prevention and cure for constipation. For cleansing the system, especially after childbirth, 'cocktails' are made with olive oil, lemon juice, honey and brandy.

Olive oil has always been treasured as a natural aid to beauty. Homer observed that the rich nobles rubbed oil daily into their skin to keep it smooth and supple. Today, Italian and other Continental beauties rub olive oil into their skin each night just as their mothers and their grandmothers did before them. The men use it too, as a body oil after baths. For luxurious, shiny hair, warm olive oil is massaged well into the scalp before a shampoo. Dry or scurfy and out-of-condition hair responds dramatically to this warm olive oil treatment, especially when wrapped for about an hour in a hot towel before washing. The more out-of-condition the hair, the longer the oil should be left on, sometimes even for the night.

When the French want an instant gleaming tan they mix olive oil with a few drops of iodine. A mixture of equal parts of olive oil and cider vinegar is a traditional remedy for sunburn. For hand care, ragged cuticles and brittle nails respond to soaking in warm olive oil.

In Spain, where olive oil is used as much as a medicine as a cooking oil, they have a saying: *'Aceite de olive todo mal quita'* which translates into English as 'Olive oil banishes every ill.'

> Herbal Medicine <

Olive oil is regarded as soothing, anti-inflammatory, laxative and stimulant to bile secretion. It is used as a safe and mild laxative, in doses up to one tablespoon, preferably taken first thing in the morning on an empty stomach. Many bowel disorders are believed to benefit from this remedy. It is recommended (in teaspoon doses) for inflamed stomach conditions, colitis and colic.

The stimulating action on bile secretion makes it useful, with other herbal medicines, in cases of gallstones and diseases of the gall bladder.

Olive leaves are used in many herbal preparations as an antispasmodic and an effective remedy against high blood pressure, and in certain heart complaints. As the leaves contain a powerful alkaloid, they should only be used as prescribed by a medical herbalist.

Olive oil is entirely beneficial. Externally it soothes pruritus and eczema and is of good value in many skin conditions. Masseuses use olive oil, often slightly warmed, to relieve stiff, arthritic or tense joints. Olive oil is regarded as a good dispersing agent which helps other medicines to be absorbed more quickly by the system.

> Culinary Use <

Olive oil reigns supreme in all Mediterranean cooking. Those of us in non-olive-growing countries can make a cheaper cooking medium by blending olive oil with sunflower or other vegetable oil.

Assuredly, salad and raw vegetable dressings taste much better made with good olive oil, but a discreet blend can be made. An old trick to improve bland oils is to soak a few chopped olives in the oil beforehand. The Romans did this to great effect. They preserved the olives in large volumes of olive oil and simply drained it off for salad dressings as needed.

A delicious long-lasting dressing is made in Greece in this way: take a handful of stoned green olives, several cloves of garlic, a pinch of cayenne pepper, a pinch of basil, and cover with a litre of pure olive oil. In a cool place this dressing will keep for months and can be strained and used when necessary. It is particularly good with winter salads and cheaper ingredients for *hors d'eouvre*.

Olives for pickling are harvested when they are green and unripe, and they remain green. Ripe olives are dark blue and turn black during pickling. Olives are pickled in brine, or, more expensively, preserved in olive oil. Modern vacuum packing keeps the fruit fresh with less preserving solution.

Green olives are used as a relish, often stuffed with nuts, anchovies, spicy red pepper, or veal forcemeat. Pickled olives are a traditional ingredient in many Italian dishes, notably antipasta and pizza. Throughout Europe, olives are eaten alone as a relish, or as an ingredient in countless *hors d'oeuvre*.

In France, olives are mixed with anchovy fillets to make anchovy butter. In country districts stoned black olives add a subtle southern flavour to *chou farci catalan* and many lamb *daubes*.

In America, Fannie Merritt Farmer of the Boston Cooking School evolved the delicious olive and almond sauce which she served with boiled or steamed fish. The sauce was made with three tablespoons of butter, three tablespoons flour, one cup (eight fluid oz) white stock, half a cup cream, quarter of a cup shredded almonds, one teaspoon beef extract, eight olives stoned and cut in quarters, one and a half teaspoons of lemon juice, a quarter of a teaspoon of salt and a few grains of cayenne pepper.

Make a roux in the usual way by melting the butter and adding the flour and white stock. Add the other ingredients gradually as the sauce thickens.

Ideally, olive oil should be stored at a cool temperature, but not in a refrigerator.

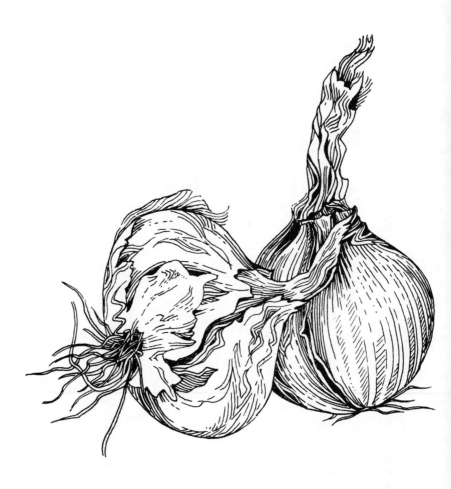

Without a doubt, onion is one of the most important vegetables and a powerful aid to health. Onion's abilities as a natural antiseptic and antibiotic have been known and valued for 5,000 years. Thanks to a team of open-minded Indian doctors, led by Dr I. S. Menon, this ancient bulb is now established as a valuable medicine.

The modern version of the onion story begins in 1968 when an article called 'Effect of Onions on Blood Fibrinolytic Activity' appeared in the *British Medical Journal*, and started with these words: 'A casual remark by a patient that in France, when a horse develops clots in the legs, it is treated by a diet of garlic and onions, led one of us to investigate onions as a possible source of a fibrinolytic agent.'

Fibrinolysis is the term which describes the ability of the blood vessels – especially veins – to dissolve the clots which can form inside them.

It is obviously vital for our bodies to prevent clotting of blood, or to get rid of any clots when they do form. Quite clearly, any food such as onion which can help the body's natural fight against clotting can fairly be described as a wonderful prevention against heart attacks and coronary disease.

The Indian doctors went on to report that they had deliberately fed groups of volunteers with fat-enriched breakfasts to which they added onions, either fried or boiled.

Normally, fatty food could be expected to lower the body's clot-preventing mechanism, but Dr Menon's group found that onions had the opposite effect. Fibrinolysis actually increased.

This important research intrigued the medical profession. Other doctors linked these findings with the fact that in parts of India, such as Rajasthan, where most of the population eat onions as a major item of their diet, coronary heart disease is much lower than in areas where, for religious reasons, onions are not eaten.

Was this coincidence, the doctors asked, or was onion a vital factor in preventing heart disease?

With interest truly aroused, further research followed thick and fast in India and Britain. This research confirmed what herbalists have believed for centuries: that in the pungent, unique smell of the onion lies its most active principles. The volatile oil and sulphurous compounds which cause the tears to run unbidden on the roughest cheeks have an equally spontaneous reaction inside the body.

At the Royal Victorian Infirmary at Newcastle upon Tyne, Dr H. A. Dewar and a team thought that the pungent taste of onion's volatile oil was a deterrent as a medicine. Dr Dewar's team isolated the odourless amino acid, cycloalliin, in onion and used this as a test in their double blind experiment with eighteen volunteers with ages ranging between 19 and 77 (eight of these people were patients with angina pectoris).

The Newcastle team found that the odourless amino acid had precisely the same clot-preventing action as whole onions.

Among the most important facts that medical research has given us about onions is one absolute boon to everyday use. It is this: when cooked in any way, baked, boiled and even fried, onions have the same effect on fibrinolytic or clot-dissolving activity. In effect, this means that we do not need to eat masses of raw onions to gain their quite remarkable protective power against heart disease.

Raw onion does contain the most powerful constituents, but it only suits strong stomachs. Incidentally, onions should never be peeled, chopped or cut long before they need to be used. Enzyme reaction starts immediately the cut surface meets the air, and raw, uncovered onion will absorb any smells in the room. The herbalist, Nicholas Culpeper, observed that 'onion doth have the power to draw corruption to it'. And an old folk use in sickrooms was to put a cut onion next to the invalid to absorb the germs. This theory is well illustrated by modern decorators' use of raw onion to soak up the smell of paint. So use only fresh cut onions or cook lightly in oil for better keeping.

Onion's other benefits are also being investigated. Some doctors believe that onion might act in a similar way on the fibrin that builds up in the inflamed joints that become such a problem in arthritis. There is some evidence to suppose that onion's particular benefits can reduce both blood sugar level and high blood pressure.

More research is needed in these areas to confirm initial findings. In the meantime, Dr Menon's research has vindicated a splendid old folk use of onion. He found that onion's powers were more marked on the older rather than the younger patient.

To the old folk, it always was an onion, more than an apple, a day that keeps the doctor away.

> Constituents <

Onion contains a volatile oil with proven antiseptic properties, the amino acid cycloalliin, sulphur compounds, pectin, flavonoid glycosides, and glucokinin. It also contains small amounts of calcium, phosphorus, potassium, iron, niacin and vitamin C. Surprisingly, one cup of cooked onions can contain more fibre than one cup of bran flakes.

> History <

The onion was one of the earliest vegetables to be cultivated and grown in the ancient civilizations of India, China and Egypt, and its use as a food plant can be traced back to 3,000 B.C. The Egyptians worshipped the onion as a sacred and medicinal plant, and it featured in many ritualistic ceremonies, especially in times of plague. It was lamented as a lost food by the Jews after their exile from Israel.

The ancient Greeks thought highly of onion. Dioscorides praised its cleansing effect. Roman doctors used many onion remedies and the Roman legions brought them north over the

Alps. Three ancient civilizations – Egypt, Rome and Greece – regarded onion as an aphrodisiac.

> Folk Use <

Traditional uses of onion are legion and varied. Onion's ancient reputation as an aphrodisiac survives in France today in the custom of taking bowls of onion soup to a young couple on their wedding night. Onion soup is regarded in France, too, as a restorative for the 'morning after'. Think of dawn at Les Halles in Paris, where market porters rub shoulders with revellers drinking onion soup.

A reputation as an aphrodisiac is very hard to prove scientifically. (The tests would be interesting, but so far government grants have not been forthcoming!) Onion's medically proven powers as an antiseptic, expectorant, diuretic, stimulant and anti-clot agent have been well observed in folk uses.

The classic folk preventative for winter colds and flu is onion soup, either standard French style or thickly chopped and cooked in milk as in Devon. A treatment for colds, coughs and tonsillitis is to pour runny honey thickly on a cut onion, cover, leave overnight. Next morning the thick syrup is taken by the spoonful. In the case of stubborn catarrh, a spoonful of horseradish is stirred into the syrup.

If researchers are divided about onion's effects on arthritis and rheumatism, folk medicine has no such doubts. Syrup of onions is used in many countries as a remedy for these complaints.

Hot onions are put on boils to bring them quickly to a head. Raw onion juice or the water onions have been cooked in is valued in Europe as a skin cleanser and complexion aid. An old anti-wrinkle preparation is made from onion juice, honey and white wax.

Instinctive folk use of onions as a heart strengthener is well established, and is vindicated by modern research. In fact French horse breeders have always fed onions to horses with a tendency to thrombosis. For heart complaints onions are taken raw, if the digestion can stand it, or eaten in very thick broths and soups.

In Spain, onion slices are poured over generously with olive oil, and eaten both as a medicine and an *hors d'oeuvre*.

> **Herbal Medicine** <

Herbalists recognize that onion has antiseptic, diuretic, eliminative, anti-spasmodic, anti-parasite and expectorant qualities.

Internationally, herbalists recommend onion remedies for coughs, colds and sore throats, particularly those which start to affect the respiratory system.

Onion stimulates digestion; it is also considered to stimulate the glands and nerves and advised in some cases of nervous exhaustion.

In Germany, the anti-parasite qualities of onion are used as a safe remedy for children with worms. Chopped onions are boiled in milk and strained and taken over one week.

Herbalists believe that the raw onion is the most powerful medicine, as its volatile oil is partially destroyed by cooking. However, raw onion is never prescribed for delicate digestions. It can cause irritation and flatulence to sensitive stomachs.

In France, where onion medicines are immensely popular, herbalists have a way of making it palatable to everyone. Onion wine is the solution. Raw onion slices are macerated (or steeped) in a mixture of white wine and honey for at least two days. The resulting liquid is strained and taken by the spoonful.

This onion wine is prescribed for rheumatism, arthritis, bronchial complaints, anaemia and exhaustion. The wine is considered a fine diuretic and used in cystitis or urinary retention. It is interesting to compare this with the old English herbals, which recommended onions steeped in Hollands gin for kidney gravel and dropsical swelling.

Raw onion poultices are applied externally for arthritis and rheumatism. Delicate skins should always be protected by grating the raw onion onto muslin or gauze.

In herbal medicine, onion is highly valued for its general protective powers against illness. Generally, it has the same power as a medicine as garlic, without being so socially devastating.

> Homeopathic medicine <

Allium cepa (onion) is a fine homeopathic remedy for certain colds. In the precise homeopathic diagnosis, *Allium cepa* is prescribed for colds with these symptoms: watery eyes, burning eyelids, sneezing, streaming nose. If there is ever any doubt about what colds will respond to *Allium cepa*, think of the common reaction to peeling an onion – running nose and eyes. Here we have an excellent example of the homeopathic law – like cures like.

Homeopathic chemists make pillules (tablets), granules and tinctures from fresh common red onion. *Allium cepa* is a standard remedy in many countries, and is recommended for every home medicine chest. The common streaming cold generally responds well to this remedy, if it is started early enough.

> Culinary Use <

An old English colloquial expression describes a wise man as one who 'knows his onions'. A wise man today chooses the onions which suit him best out of the several hundred varieties available. Fortunately, all onions share the medicinal active principles. A good rule of thumb is: the stronger the smell and flavour, the more powerful and active the constituents. It is not so easy to make a similar rule about colour and strength. Spanish onions with their golden brown skins are mild, but in some hot countries brown-skinned onions are too strong to eat raw. It depends on the climate.

The tear-jerking substance in onion only gets active when a

bulb is cut. (Whole, sound onions have hardly any smell.) All sorts of ideas are put forward as preventions against tearful chopping of onions; one quite effective one is to peel the outer layers off under a running cold tap. Since enzyme reaction is responsible for the tears, some people inhibit this by putting the onion in the refrigerator for a while before chopping.

Milder onions are much better raw and in salads. Two popular varieties are:

1. The Welsh onion (or ciboule) which does not form true bulbs and whose long green leaves are used very much like chives. This variety, so popular in America and Japan, is, in fact, native to Siberia and has nothing to do with Wales at all. 'Welsh' is a corruption of the German *welsche*, meaning foreign.

2. The Egyptian (or tree) onion, a curious variety which grows a cluster of bulbs on top of one-metre-high stems instead of flowers. It is very good for small gardens. As the bulbs are so neat and regular in size it is often used in pickling or in onion dishes where presentation is important.

Small pearl bunching onions are specially cultivated for pickling. Chives, shallots, leeks and garlic are all members of the *Allium* family and share common factors.

Onions are valued as an incomparable condiment and flavouring in regional cuisine ranging from Hindu to Greek. The flexibility of this vegetable defies imagination. It can be baked, boiled, fried, stuffed, braised, pickled, puréed or glazed, as well as being the usual base for stews, soups and casseroles.

In Greece, a pleasant onion dish is made with small, uniform onions cooked slowly in *court bouillon* or white wine and water and served either as a starter or as part of the main course.

According to Apicius, a favourite Roman dish consisted of onions mixed with pounded celery seed and fresh lettuce leaves. Another inventive Apicius recipe was stuffed fish rolls with onion sauce. Unfortunately, Apicius considered porpoise a delicacy and just right for onion sauce, but this ancient dish is very good today with white cod or cheaper fish that needs imaginative flavouring. Apicius blended the fish with oregano, parsley, coriander, cumin and dried mint, shaped it into rissoles, fried them in oil, and served them with a delicate onion sauce flavoured with lovage and savory.

By the way, don't throw away lovely golden onion skins. Wash them, and add them to your soups and stews for a fine natural colouring.

> PAPAYA <
(papaw or paw paw)

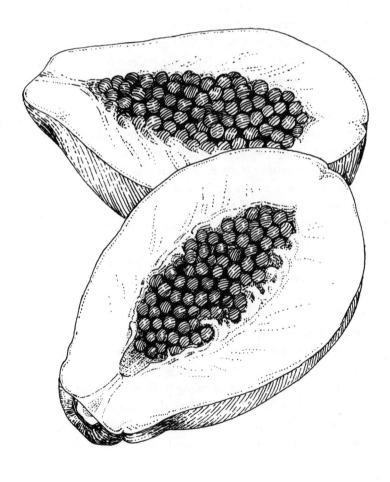

Papaw (or paw paw) is the popular name for this delicious fruit which has such remarkable benefits. Every part of the papaya tree has value, but the full-grown *unripe* fruit yields a milky latex called papain which is greatly valued by modern medicine.

Papain contains several interesting enzymes which have an astonishing effect on the digestive process. Its action closely resembles pepsin, the enzyme in the stomach which breaks up protein for digestion.

Consider this: papain is capable of digesting 35 times its own weight of lean meat or 300 times its own weight of egg albumen. One of the enzymes acts on fat, another on milk.

From this it is clear to see how papain can help us in many problems of digestion, such as heartburn, dyspepsia, bloating and anti-social gas or wind.

The enzymes in papain have proved that they can act swiftly on meat, milk and eggs. What an invaluable aid in this stressful age of quick eating. Many of us bolt our food and do not have the time or the teeth to chew each mouthful. Anxious or incomplete digestion then causes havoc and restless nights.

Officially, papain is recognized as a medicine not only for its protein-digesting qualities but also because it deals with excessive mucus in the mouth and stomach.

Pure papain is made into a variety of tablets and preparations by the pharmaceutical industry, and prescribed for many digestive troubles. Health food or other specialist shops also sell papain tablets and powders.

The golden, ripe papaya has its own qualities. Ripe fruit is not as potent as the unripe fruit, but it does contain many specific benefits.

One aspect of ripe papaya's healing properties hit the headlines in 1977 when doctors at Guy's Hospital, London, used the fresh fruit after a kidney operation. The patient had developed an infection which refused to respond to modern drugs. Dr

Christopher Rudge remembered that in the South African bush he had seen tribesmen cure wounds and ulcers with papaya fruit. A poultice of pulped fruit was applied, almost as a last resort. The infection healed quickly. Many of the doctors were surprised, and one commented: 'It worked, but we don't know why.'

Had the news reached the shores of the Caribbean or the tribesmen in the veldt, there would have been no surprise at all.

> Constituents <

Papain (the dried latex of the unripe fruit) is a rich source of proteolytic enzymes. The seeds contain a glucoside caricin and myrosin which together produce a volatile oil like mustard. Papaya leaves contain an alkaloid, carpaine.

The ripe fruit contains free amino acids, enzymes, fibre, potassium, calcium, iron and excellent amounts of vitamin C and vitamin A.

> History <

The early explorers were intrigued by the unknown and exotic papaya tree which was so revered in its native habitat. Christopher Columbus was deeply impressed when he saw the natives of the Caribbean eating vast heavy meals of meat and fish without any apparent discomfort provided that the banquet also included papaya.

Marco Polo credited papaya with saving the lives of his crew when they were badly stricken with scurvy. The fruit's rich vitamin C content treated the scurvy while the pulp cured their festering sores.

Ponce de Leon noted that the natives called the papaya tree by many names which translated meant 'keep well' or 'fruit of health'. Vasco da Gama called it the Golden Tree of Life.

> Folk Use <

All the romance of tropical folk lore is evoked by the dusky golden papaya. In the Caribbean it is still 'the medicine tree', and the 'fruit of health'.

Indeed, the people go to the papaya tree much as Western civilization reaches for its medicine chest. They use the raw unripe juice for any digestive ailment and as a system cleanser; the seeds are chewed for heart complaints; the ripe fruit is applied to cleaned wounds and sores; the leaves are wrapped around tough meat and fowl to tenderize them in cooking.

How interesting it would be to plot the development of folk use as the papaya was taken from its native tropical America to Australia, South America, Africa, Tanzania, Hawaii and the U.S.A.

In Africa, papaya juice is gargled for sore throats and inflamed gums. Mexicans rub the fruit on boils, pimples, warts and corns. Polynesian islanders mix fresh papaya into cough medicine.

Despite the cultural differences, there is a deep ethnic understanding of the power of papaya to heal wounds and sores and aid ailing digestions.

Wherever the papaya tree grows, the women make great use of the fruit as a beauty treatment. Cosmetic firms spend millions advertising products that can lift dead cells and treat dry skin. Papaya pulp is quietly used for exactly the same reason and with effect. It is rubbed over flaky skins or scurvy scalps with dandruff. Even non-problem skins are regularly rubbed with papaya slices to keep them springy and lustrous.

In the papaya, nature has been judicious as well as bountiful, for the ripe fruit is considered an aid to male fertility.

> Herbal Medicine <

Papain is recognized as one of the finest digestive aids known. It is used in herbal medicines in much the same way as orthodox medicines and prescribed for the same problems, indigestion, dyspepsia and flatulence. Herbalists also use papain tablets and the ripe fruit to treat disorders of fat digestion, gall bladder and liver problems. Papaya juice is recommended for cases of croup and sore throat. It can be rubbed over warts and corns. As a system cleanser, ripe papaya juice is taken in wine-glass amounts several times a day for at least four days, or it can be alternated with pineapple and beet juice. Juice from the green, unripe papaya is valued as a rejuvenator and used in cases of premature ageing.

> **Culinary Use** <

Fresh papaya may be served either as a starter, like melon, or as a dessert, perfect in its own right. It is good in fruit cocktails, fruit salads, sherbets, syllabubs, preserves, marmalade or jam.

Papain is a most effective meat tenderizer and is used in high technology by the meat industry. In the Caribbean, cooks place a layer of papaya pulp over tough meat and achieve succulent results. You can transform cheaper cuts of meat in this way or make liver and offal acceptable to even the most critical children.

Papaya salt can be bought as a tenderizer and is often included in barbecue seasonings. Papaya juice can be bought commercially or bottled at home. It is subject to quick fermentation, but this can be overcome by adding a few drops of glycerine.

> PARSLEY <

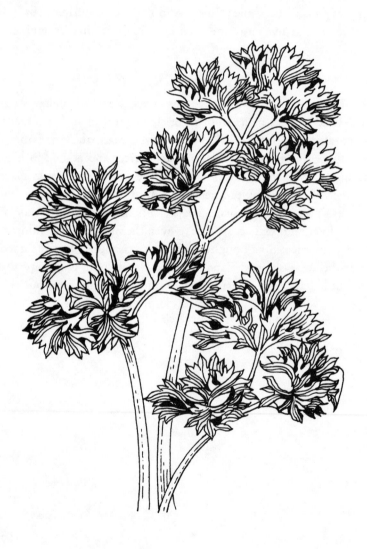

Parsley has been known for centuries as a green kitchen herb and widely appreciated for its medicinal values. Parsley is rich in vitamins and minerals and contains many powerfully active constituents.

It is sad to see this fine medicinally potent food used as a mere sprig limply garnishing the main meal, when it is more health giving than many dishes it decorates. One herb expert is fond of saying that too often people push aside the parsley decoration uneaten and tuck into the food underneath when, for their health's sake, they would do better to push away the food and eat the parsley.

Parsley has several essential, volatile oils. One of these oils, apiol, is a strong drug which can be dangerous in large or distilled amounts. It was formerly used widely in the treatment of malaria and fevers.

Herbalists have a long tradition of using parsley and its essential oils in medicines, with discretion, to treat many illnesses. Parsley's volatile oils promote the blood circulation in the pelvic regions. The combination of active constituents in parsley is known to act strongly on the uterus, which is the reason why large amounts should never be taken by pregnant women. This herb's actions can be valuable in regulating menstruation and relieving the uncomfortable water retention and swelling that is so bothersome to many women just before and during monthly periods.

In other ways, too, parsley is an effective medicine. It is a diuretic which greatly assists the kidneys to function regularly and resist disease. For this reason it is widely used in alternative medicine to treat inflammation of the kidneys and bladder.

For the stomach, parsley acts as a carminative and relieves flatulence, and generally aids digestion.

This beneficial herb is also a natural deodorizer and acts as an instant breath sweetener after spicy foods or cigarettes.

Traditionally, parsley sprigs are vigorously chewed after eating garlic to take the smell away from the breath.

> Constituents <

Parsley contains essential oil with apiol, flavone glycoside apiin, myristicene, pinene and other terpenes, fatty oil with petroselinic acid.

Parsley is rich in vitamins A and C. It also provides good amounts of iron, potassium, calcium, and the B vitamins thiamine, riboflavin and niacin.

> History <

The ancient Greeks had a saying, 'They are at the parsley and rue' – meaning that a project had barely begun, since these herbs were planted in thick borders at the edge of flower beds.

In fact, the Greeks held parsley in superstitious awe, and would never bring it to the table. According to their legend, the mythological hero Archemorus was carelessly laid by his nurse on a parsley leaf and was eaten by serpents. Henceforth, parsley became the herb of oblivion.

Plutarch described how a Greek army on the march met some donkeys loaded with parsley. The soldiers panicked with fright, dropping their weapons and fleeing despite the curses of their officers.

Somewhat contrarily, the Greeks also crowned the victors of the Isthmian games with parsley chaplets, and wove it into garlands for special feasts. Theocritus painted the image vividly:

> At Sparta's palace twenty beauteous mayds
> The pride of Greece, fresh garlands crowned their heads
> With hyacinths and twining parsley drest
> Graced joyful Menelaus' marriage feast.

The Romans thought that parsley caused sterility in women and forbade it to those of child-bearing age. On the other hand, they were keen observers of the herb's nutritional riches and fed it to soldiers and gladiators before fights to make them strong. At Roman banquets, sprigs of parsley were worn around the neck to ward off intoxication.

Many fascinating stories and legends have been woven around parsley. The seed is notoriously difficult to germinate, and it is said to thrive in the garden only if the woman is the boss of the household. Tradition says that out of every seven rows of parsley planted, six will promptly go to the devil.

> Folk Use <

The old herbalists held parsley in high esteem, and this has obviously influenced folk usage throughout the centuries.

'Water of Parcelly' was among the usual still-room products of Tudor households. William Turner wrote in 1551: 'If Parsley is thrown into fish ponds it will heal the sick fishes therein.'

Nicholas Culpeper was a firm advocate of parsley:

It is very comfortable to the stomach . . . good for wind and to remove obstructions both of the liver and spleen . . . the seed is effectual to break the stone and ease the pains and torments thereof . . . the leaves of parsley laid to the eyes that are inflammed with heat or swollen, relieves them if it be used with bread or meat.

Parsley is traditionally valued as a kind herb to women. It is taken infused as a tea (one teaspoon of chopped leaves to one cup of boiling water) to regulate menstruation and relieve the cramp-like pains that sometimes occur. Poultices made from parsley leaves steeped in vinegar are laid on sore breasts. In the old days, wet nurses used parsley to keep their breasts healthy.

Cellulite, that unpleasant 'orange-peel' skin, cannot fairly be said to be an all-female problem. Plump men get it too, especially round the tops of the thighs. Parsley tea is a folk remedy for cellulite, both drunk normally and applied to the skin as a lotion.

Standard parsley tea is allowed to stand for at least seven

hours, then strained and rubbed into the scalp to stimulate the growth of hair, discourage head lice, and cure dandruff. It is also a standard folk remedy for preventing and treating baldness in men. When used externally as a lotion in this way much stronger brews can be made from the crushed seeds of parsley.

In Holland, the bruised seeds are made into ointment with fresh, unsalted butter to treat ringworm. This ointment, or warm parsley tea, is used to soothe all sorts of insect bites and stings, especially those which swell up.

These soothing qualities are used with great effect in conjunctivitis or for generally bleary eyes. Decoct or boil two teaspoons of clean chopped leaves for six minutes, allow to cool until just warm, strain, and apply as a cold compress on cotton wool.

In France, fresh parsley and garlic sandwiches are eaten in the winter to prevent colds. The digestant properties of the herb are valued greatly in France. Rich meals of *foie gras* or other epicurean delights are often finished off with parsley tea 'for the stomach'.

As a beauty aid, parsley has a long and interesting folk usage. It was perhaps the first deodorant. Bunches of parsley were rubbed underneath the armpits to remove perspiration and freshen up the body.

For the face, parsley cuts down on oily skin and adds a lustrous gleam to the complexion. It is too harsh to rub directly on the skin, so always use parsley juice or the lotion as brewed from standard parsley tea, steeped for 15 minutes. Add this lotion also to the final rinse when shampooing, to give a fine sheen to your hair.

> **Herbal Medicine** <

Parsley is used as one of the regular kidney tonics which are so valued for prevention as well as cure. The more powerful roots or seed are generally used herbally, but a standard parsley tea is also effective. Use one teaspoon of the dried herb to one cup of boiling water.

Herbalists make an excellent kidney tonic by mixing dried

parsley root with the roots of celery, asparagus and fennel. These dried roots are readily available from herbal suppliers or health food shops. Measure out approximately two teaspoons of dried root into a non-aluminium pan. Pour on 500ml water, bring to the boil for one minute, then transfer to a warm teapot to stand or infuse for a few minutes. Strain, and take one wineglassful of this mixture with a few drops of lemon juice before each meal for two or three days consecutively.

One leading herbalist believes that this kidney tonic, taken every three months, should keep most people free from chronic kidney diseases and infections.

Herbally, parsley is seen as an insurance policy against bladder and kidney diseases. The action of parsley as a stimulant on the uterus is used in herbal medicines to treat many menstrual disorders.

Parsley medicines are also used to treat rheumatism and to eliminate excess body fluids.

Whenever parsley is taken as a medicine, it must be borne in mind that it is a powerful drug in concentrated doses. Obviously, parsley is quite safe to use generously as a fresh herb, but concentrated doses should not be taken for more than a few days at a time, and never by pregnant women. To throw a little more light on this one can say that parsley tea made from the fresh or dried herb is much less strong than decoctions made from the root or seed of the plant.

> **Culinary Use** <

Here is one of the most popular and widely grown kitchen herbs, essential in many recipes for flavour and decoration. There are four main varieties: curly-leaved parsley with its crinkly, deeply divided leaves; flat-leaved parsley, so popular in Europe; Hamburg parsley, cultivated for its long tapering root which tastes rather like parsnip; Neapolitan or celery-leaved parsley, grown specially for its stems.

Parsley has so many fine qualities as a medicinal herb and a flavouring that it should be treated with great respect. Forget about those sprigs of parsley sitting on the top of grilled fish or meat dishes. Use parsley with dash and verve like the French chefs.

In French they have a term – *persiller* – which means to sprinkle a dish with chopped parsley. A *persillade* is the culinary term for chopped parsley, often mixed with chopped garlic or shallots, which is added to dishes at the end of cooking. This *persillade* greatly improves the flavour and, of course, retains the medicinal value of parsley itself. Often meat is sautéed in butter or oil and sprinkled with *persillade,* as in *persillade de boeuf.* Cold or left over meat can be quite transformed in this way. There is no doubt that finely chopped parsley, garlic or shallots greatly improve the appearance and taste of many dishes. Parsley is also used in many sauces, such as tartare, vinaigrette, ravigote and verte.

Bear in mind that parsley stalks are stronger than the leaves. European cooks use parsley leaves lavishly, but they chop them very finely indeed, and this seems to distribute the flavours most equably. A huge variety of European dishes are flavoured with chopped parsley – soup, fish, shellfish, meat, poultry and salads. Watch an Italian chopping parsley to sprinkle on his minestrone. You might think he was trying to split the atom.

Parsley should be well washed to get rid of any grit, then wrung dry in kitchen paper. Unfortunately, as a dried herb, parsley loses much of its flavour and texture. It is actually one of the few herbs which do not respond to the usual herb drying treatment. As a compensation, however, it freezes remarkably well. So chop up washed parsley leaves finely and freeze them, with a little water, in an ice cube tray. Prise out the frozen chunks into a freezer bag and add a dash of soda water to keep them separate. Frozen parsley cubes retain their freshness well enough to use as garnishes or decoration, and are an ideal addition to soups, stocks and casseroles.

When using mixed herbs, a sprig of parsley is always part of the *bouquet garni,* and finely chopped parsley is the main ingredient of a *fines herbes* mixture. Parsley is the main ingredient in *beurre maître d'hôtel,* more commonly known as parsley butter. This is delicious with lightly boiled potatoes, or carrots. The secret in making parsley butter is to mix it in a *warm* bowl. Allow about one and a half tablespoons of parsley to 50 grams of butter. Mash with a fork and add a few drops of lemon juice.

Parsley butter or parsley sauce, made in the usual way with a basic roux, is an invaluable addition to vegetarian cookery, and can transform a dish of elderly vegetables.

❯ PINEAPPLE ❮

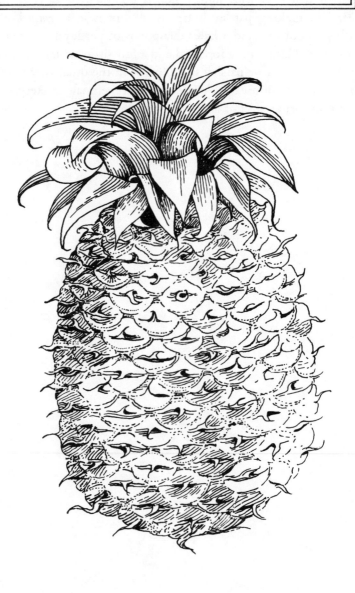

> Health <

The exquisite tasting pineapple contains an enzyme rather like the better-known papain in papaya. Pineapple's enzyme is called bromelin, sometimes spelt bromelain in the U.S.A. Like papain, it also has the power to split protein, thus providing a very valuable natural digestive aid.

Bromelin does differ from papain, and more chemical study is needed to understand its complex reactions fully. There is one difference which can be appreciated straight away. It is the unripe papaya which provides the valuable enzymes, but ripening does not destroy the bromelin in pineapple.

A fresh pineapple is an excellent aid to health. It is well worth buying fresh pineapples, even in countries where the fruit is an expensive import. Enzymes are destroyed by temperatures of over 140°F. (60°C.), so canned or bottled juice cannot have the healing properties of the fresh fruit. Frozen juice, on the other hand, does retain some enzyme action.

Bromelin enzyme is freeze-dried and used medically to treat swelling, internal inflammation, and to accelerate tissue repair. Bromelin is an effective natural healer – not only does it help damaged tissues, it also has a soothing effect on the stomach and greatly improves the digestion of meat and other proteins.

However, this interesting enzyme has some unusual actions. It prevents gelatine from 'jelling' and clots milk, so pineapple milk shakes are not really a good use of this beneficial fruit.

Pineapple is believed to have a good effect on relieving mucus, but research on this has been inconclusive. However, tests in Britain in 1978 showed that a weekly course of fresh juice once a month could help women with painful periods of menstruation.

The bromelin enzyme has been medically proved to be active against sore or 'furry' throats, a fine vindication of the old folk use of pineapple juice.

> Constituents <

As well as bromelin, pineapple contains good amounts of potassium, calcium, phosphorus and sulphur and moderate amounts of iron, fibre and the vitamins A and C, with a trace of B vitamin.

> History <

The botanical name *Ananas* is the name given to the fruit by the American Indians, and it has been adopted as the common name in practically all European languages except English.

Pineapple is native to tropical South America and was introduced to North America, tropical Asia and Africa and the Malayan archipelago. The pineapple grows well in hot countries and especially fine fruits now come from Hawaii and Australia.

In colder countries, the pineapple was considered a rare exotic delicacy for centuries. King Charles II was painted stiffly holding the first pineapple ever grown in England. His gardener, Rose, claimed to have grown the fruit in the Royal greenhouses, but it was more likely to have been secretly imported from America.

> Folk Use <

In the warm countries where pineapple grows naturally, it is greatly valued as an instant medicine.

In Hawaii, pineapple juice is a popular cure for dyspepsia and indigestion. People inclined to stomach troubles regularly finish a meal with fresh pineapple slices.

Throughout the tropics, pineapple juice is drunk or gargled as a standard remedy for sore throats, preferably at the first sign of soreness.

Crushed or pulped fruit is put on bruises or swellings and also used as a regular complexion aid. Like papaya, pineapple can remove dead tissue and bring colour and suppleness to the skin. In Africa, pineapple slices are rubbed all over the body as a skin toner and freshener. Corns or hardened patches of skin are rubbed with pineapple daily. Juice is taken, too, when the appetite is jaded.

> Herbal Medicine <

Pineapple juice is considered an outstanding treatment for stomach complaints where there is any inflammation present. It is prescribed as a specific for peptic ulcers, chronic gastritis, catarrh, colitis, and enteritis. For these conditions, a wine glass of pineapple juice is recommended to be sipped slowly before each meal.

Before antibiotics, pineapple juice was given as a treatment for tuberculosis and diphtheria.

Herbalists advise fresh pineapple during bronchitis and all sore throats.

> Culinary Use <

Pineapple is so delicious and beneficial that it is far better eaten fresh than cooked. It can be used in cold desserts like sorbets or sherbets without losing nutritional value, but remember, it will not 'jell'.

When pineapples are to be exported, they are often picked green and allowed to ripen on the journey. Such pineapples are markedly less sweet than fruit which has been allowed to ripen naturally.

Before eating, a pineapple should be trimmed of its crown, rind and centre of the fruit which becomes woody. For this reason, slices of pineapple are ring-shaped. (Although, when pineapples are expensive, people are inclined to eat the woody centre and all.)

Pineapple has a tenderizing effect on meat similar to that of papaya. A layer of chopped pineapple can make tough or cheaper cuts of meat succulent and tender. The American quick grill of a slice of gammon or ham topped with pineapple is both a tasty meal and a good digestive aid.

> **POTATO** <

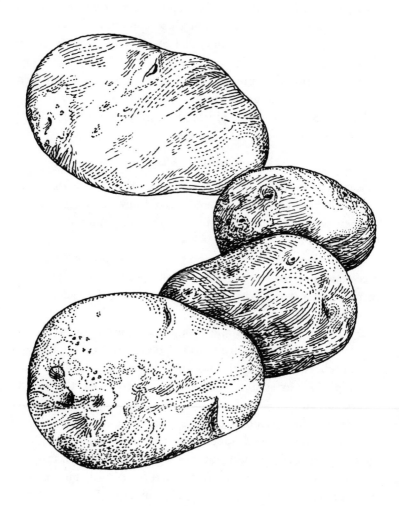

The common or garden potato is actually a dramatic vegetable. It belongs to the *Solanaceae* botanical family which includes deadly nightshade, tobacco, thorn apple and tomato, as well as some of the most notorious herbs in the history of medicine. Many of the group have been used to soothe pain or induce oblivion since the earliest times. In China today, the thorn apple is used as an anaesthetic by orthodox surgeons.

Potato's leaves and berries share toxic alkaloids with its first cousin, deadly nightshade, and should never be eaten. The tuber beneath the soil is what we all know as potato and is entirely wholesome. The narcotic properties of the nightshades only develop on contact with light, which is why good gardeners earth up the crop. When young tubers come into contact with light they can turn green and develop a poisonous substance, solanin. So cut out all the green skin on potatoes, or better still, don't accept them from the greengrocer.

It is worth while making the point that discoloured, damaged or diseased potatoes should never be bought, or should be tossed out promptly. In 1972 Sir James Renwick put forward the theory that blighted potatoes eaten during the first month of pregnancy may cause spina bifida and other defects.

Buy fresh, sound potatoes and use them generously, for there is evidence that this vegetable is a good dietary weapon against heart disease.

Potatoes are rich in vegetable fibre. Research at Belfast University has shown that potato fibre has the same cholesterol-reducing ability as bran fibre.

In 1975, in another fascinating Irish study, 1,154 pairs of Irish brothers who had both grown up in Ireland were studied by researchers after one brother had emigrated to the U.S.A. The stay-at-home Irish brothers actually ate *more* animal fat but had the same cholesterol levels. Other variable factors, such as smoking, sugar, protein and cholesterol intake were carefully controlled. The major difference in the survey was that the Irish brothers ate lots of potatoes and averaged 6.4 grams of fibre a day, whereas the American brothers only ate 3.6 grams of fibre a day, mostly as fruit and vegetables. At the end of the project, researchers found that the American brothers had developed a massive 90 per cent more heart disease than the Irish brothers.

The high potassium content of potato might be another clue to its benefit to the heart. Other studies in the U.S.A. have shown that patients with a low blood potassium and low potassium intake are more susceptible generally to heart disease.

How sad, then, that the potato is often the first thing cut out of a menu by dieters and slimmers. At first glance, it is high in calories, but we do not yet know how many of these calories are unabsorbable natural fibre which passes straight through the body in the way nature intended.

In yet another Irish study, volunteers were given one pound of potatoes to eat each day. They could eat anything else they liked at all, but they must eat one pound of potatoes. After a few weeks nearly all the volunteers had lost weight and suffered none of the empty or irritable symptoms of usual dieting. The conclusion was that the potatoes were so filling that the dieters did not crave other foods.

In Germany, the *kartoffeln* diet is immensely popular with slimmers. There are several variations on this diet, but basically, potatoes are eaten twice a day (without butter, of course) and the water in which the potatoes have boiled is drunk as a beverage. Grated fresh vegetables and salads, white fish, and occasional lean meat are the foods which are eaten with the potatoes, and the diet kept up for about two weeks. No bread is eaten during this period.

The old wives' tale that the goodness of potato lies 'just beneath the skin' may have some justification because of the physical way in which the tuber develops. Potatoes provide proteins, minerals such as iron, calcium, and the vitamins B and

C, which are not present in such significant quantities in other carbohydrate foods. The vitamin C varies according to variety, but most especially according to season. There is most vitamin C in new potatoes and least in late winter. The vitamin value is lowest in potatoes that have been peeled thickly, boiled in too much water and kept hot or reheated before serving. A medium-sized potato supplies an average of 33 milligrams of vitamin C, or about the same amount as a glass of tomato juice, and 1.5 milligrams of iron, the amount in an egg. In the winter, potatoes may be the chief source of these vitamins for families in poor regions.

The highest nutritive value obviously comes from eating the potatoes in their skins. They are easy to scrub clean under a running tap or in a bowl of water with a stiff dish-cleaning brush set aside especially for the purpose. Really keen health food fans put their potatoes in the fridge for a while before cutting and cooking them, to inhibit the enzyme action when the cut surface is exposed to the air. In this way loss of vitamin C is prevented.

The real sin in preparing potatoes is to peel them early in the morning and leave them swimming in cold water at room temperature while the family goes off to church or ice-skating at the weekends. Yet many efficient housewives feel they are getting ahead by pre-preparing potatoes in this way. One nutritionist has commented that you might as well drink the water and throw the potatoes away. If potatoes must be peeled in advance, put them in a plastic bag in the refrigerator without added moisture. Heat them as quickly as possible and use all the liquid for stocks.

> **Constituents** <

Potatoes contain iron, protein, calcium, good amounts of vitamin B and C, and excellent amounts of potassium. They provide energy in the form of carbohydrate; two and a half per cent of non-water content is vegetable fibre.

According to popular legend, Sir Walter Raleigh introduced the potato to England and Europe from Virginia in North America. He is supposed to have eaten the new vegetable enthusiastically, but unfortunately chose the berries and leaves and was violently sick. Sir Walter ordered the 'noxious plant' to be rooted up and thrown away, but in doing so his Irish gardener discovered the wholesome tubers under the soil and propagated them secretly. The Irish certainly accepted the potato long before the rest of Europe.

Some historians credit Sir John Hawkins with the introduction of the potato. You can take your choice from these glamorous Elizabethans. There is sound evidence to suppose that *Solanum tuberosum* is indigenous to Peru and was taken from there to Virginia and thence to Europe. The first European potato was grown in Spain in about 1580. Another Irish connection occurred when the ships of the Armada foundered on the west coast of Ireland – the peasants plundered the stores and carried off potato tubers which they planted along the coast of Kerry and Cork.

The American colonists quickly realized the value of the potato, while the Irish elevated it to a national dish, but nearly 200 years went by before the new vegetable became a field crop in England. There were years of famine and high corn prices, but the nutritious potato which could have saved the poor from starvation or scurvy was fiercely opposed.

The Puritans were suspicious of the potato because it was not mentioned in the Bible and greatly feared it might 'provoke lust'. Francis Bacon praised it as a health-giving and fortifying food, to little avail. William Cobbett, for reasons best known to himself, railed against 'Ireland's lazy root', as he called the potato, and described Sir Walter Raleigh as 'one of the greatest villains upon earth, who ... [they say] first brought this root to England'.

In Germany there was a terrible famine during the reign of

Frederick the Great, and he sent wagons loaded with potatoes to Kolberg. The starving citizens sent them back with an indignant message: 'These things have neither taste nor smell. Not even the dogs would eat them. What good are they to us?'

In spite of this, by the mid-eighteenth century potatoes had become a staple in the diet of the urban and rural poor throughout northern Europe. So much so that the devastating potato crop disease in the next century altered the course of history. In *The Englishman's Food*, Professor Sir Jack Drummond commented:

The food situation in 1845 became desperate for the very poor as a result of a widespread invasion of 'potato disease' in conjunction with a poor corn harvest. England has never been nearer to revolution. The fungus (*Phytophtora infestans*), however, did what twenty years of bitter agitation had failed to do: it brought about the repeal of the Corn Laws in 1846.

In Ireland, two years of potato disease were followed by the potato famine of 1847 and caused the mass migration which so influenced the growth of America.

Ironically enough, when potatoes were first brought from the New World they were known as 'Virginian' potatoes; now in the United States they are often called 'Irish' potatoes.

> ## > Folk Use <

Some of the folk uses of the potato can fairly be called quaint. One very old English remedy against rheumatism was to carry a raw potato on one's person. Ladies in Georgian times even had special pockets made for their potatoes in their beautiful, elaborate dresses. An Irish solution for a sore throat was to wear a boiled potato in a woollen sock around the neck. In France, a small raw potato was carried against sciatica and lumbago and replaced the moment it dried out. In many country districts today these old potato remedies are still widely used.

However, many of the well-established uses show that the folk have a fine appreciation of the medicinal powers of the potato. Centuries before the authorities had worked out a preventative for scurvy, people were instinctively using potatoes for their anti-scorbutic powers.

Long before limes and lemons were adopted by the Navy, sailors crammed as many potatoes as possible into their knapsacks and ate them raw as a prevention against the dreaded 'voyage sickness'.

Raw potato juice is still a popular remedy against rheumatism and gout in many countries, including America, England, Russia, France and Germany. A potato is juiced, or finely chopped to express the juice which is sipped throughout the day. It can taste rather fierce and is better flavoured with carrot or other pleasant raw vegetables.

Hot potato water (as hot as can be borne) is used externally for swollen and painful rheumatoid joints, and in sciatica and lumbago.

The Romanies, too, use potato juice for rheumatism. They value it also for stomach upsets, and rub raw potato slices on the skin to improve and soften it.

Grated raw potato poultice is used internationally to relieve the pain from minor scalds and burns, especially sunburn. Raw grated potato or potato juice applied straight away to sunburnt areas is very soothing.

In the Soviet Union, raw potato slices are placed over swollen, puffy or sore eyes, and rubbed over chilblains. Raw potato is widely used in folklore beauty treatment for normal or oily skin. It is reputed to be healing and good for eczema.

> Herbal Medicine <

According to the English herb authority, Mrs Maud Grieve, the folk uses of raw potato juice for rheumatism and gout have a scientific basis. In herbal treatment today, raw potato juice would be a dietary adjunct to other herbal medicines. The raw juice is taken in tablespoon amounts before meals.

Naturopaths believe that raw potato juice is good for acid conditions and rheumatism. Raw potato is also recommended for skin complaints. The juice is drunk throughout the day, and applied cold externally as a lotion.

Potato juice therapy is popular with European herbalists who use it to treat rheumatic and lumbago-type complaints and also certain gastric conditions. They apply hot fomentations made from potato juice to swollen, rheumatic limbs, followed by massage with embrocation.

Those who find raw potato juice unpalatable will certainly be able to tolerate the water the potatoes have cooked in.

> Culinary Use <

Potato is such a tried and true basic that it is often left out of the more imaginative dishes. In day-to-day cooking it is automatic to think in terms of meat, potatoes and two veg or steak and chips. Why? If the potato were a rare vegetable it would be treated as an exotic and presented in pride of place.

That is not to mock the basic potato, far from it. The common potato can reach heights that would satisfy Brillat-Savarin. A good cook can turn mashed potatoes into ambrosian delights. The potatoes are lighter and fluffier if *hot* milk is used. Some people heat the milk and butter or polyunsaturated margarine in a saucepan before beating it well into the potato. In restaurants this mixture is then forced into piping bags to create fancy shapes.

Many of our basic potato dishes are adapted from French cuisine, which has hundreds of cooking methods. The French have given us Duchess potatoes, Dauphine potatoes, potato croquettes, potato fondantes, potato cakes and macaire potatoes. In one notable case it was the old culture's turn to learn from the new world. *Pommes frites* in France today are very influenced by

American french fries (the equivalent of English chips), an interesting cross-fertilization of ideas.

Because potatoes are such a cheap staple food, many of the more imaginative recipes come out of regional cookery books. In Wales, *punch-nep* is made by boiling equal quantities of potato and white turnip separately, then mashing them both well together with butter, seasoning with salt and pepper. The mixture is then packed tightly into a dish, and prodded with holes into which is poured sour cream. Yogurt would certainly do instead. Stelk is an old English supper dish made from winter potatoes and spring onions. The onions are trimmed into half-inch lengths including the green tops, and simmered in a pan of milk. The flavoured milk is strained on to the cooked potatoes to mash them with. Finally the onion pieces are forked in to make a green, tasty dish which improves tired old potatoes and goes well with salads or cold meat.

American colonial cookery developed O'Brion potatoes in which a gadget similar to a melon scoop is used to make neat balls. These were fried and served with cooked onions and pimentoes and finely chopped parsley.

In the Ukraine, new potatoes are most welcome after the long hard winter and are made into a festive dish with Smetana sauce with green onion and paprika. Smetana sauce is made by bringing two cups of thick, sour cream to the boil and adding half a cup of chopped green onions, then simmering very slowly, uncovered, for about 30 to 40 minutes until the flavours are developed.

Coeliacs and others who need to exclude gluten (found in wheat, oats, barley and rye) totally from their diet search avidly for unusual potato recipes to add variety to their diet.

There are about 1,600 varieties of potato in common use around the world. Generally, potatoes are closer textured and waxier in the early part of the season, becoming mealier and more floury towards the end. Variety is important but the season is also relevant. Potato varieties can be matched exactly to each dish and good cooks make full use of the wide choice available. If in doubt, the Potato Marketing Board is only too happy to send explanatory leaflets and suggestions for the many varieties.

Potatoes should be kept in a cool place, away from light. The ideal temperature for storage is between 50°F. (10°C.) and 60°F. (16°C.). Too high a temperature causes potatoes to sprout and shrivel. At too low a temperature the potato develops a sweet flavour. Unwashed potatoes keep better than washed.

> SAGE <

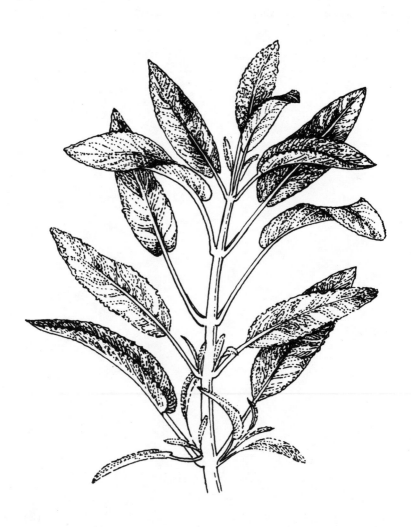

> Health <

The botanical name for sage is translated variously as 'to save', 'to heal', or 'I am well'. Certainly this herb is widely appreciated for its medicinal values and is traditionally believed to promote longevity. In country districts throughout Europe people still chew a few leaves of sage every morning, perhaps heeding the motto: 'Who has sage in his garden he would live for aye.' Interestingly enough, sage contains a substance called ketone thujone which helps animal tissues to resist putrefaction.

Sage also contains volatile oils and other medicinally active ingredients which are naturally antiseptic and stimulant. In tea made from the dried leaves the medicinal substances are still active, and have been shown to lower blood sugar levels in diabetics. Sage tea is a classic treatment for sore or relaxed throats and bleeding gums. Until quite recently sage was listed in the United States Pharmocopoeia as a remedy for inflamed sore throats, tonsillitis and ulcerated mouth conditions.

The stimulating properties of sage are valuable for long-standing fatigue and after illnesses.

> Constituents <

Sage contains volatile oils, tannin, resin and ketone thujone.

> History <

Sage is native to the Mediterranean but it is now grown medicinally right throughout the world, even as far away as China. The Roman legions took sage with them to colder climes where its virtues were quickly appreciated.

The Greeks made great use of sage medicines and almost created a ceremony of picking the herb. They believed that it was most effective when it was picked on May the first before sunrise. Dioscorides recommended sage as a remedy for most kidney troubles, rheumatism, ulcers, consumption, coughs and sore throats. He closely observed his patients when they were taking sage medicine, and claimed to have discovered the fact that sage can restore the colour to fading black hair.

> Folk Use <

According to folk medicine, sage has a regulating effect on the hormones and is always given to girls in puberty, pregnant women and those with menopausal problems. This long traditional use may date back to the Romans, who advocated sage for pregnant women or for those who found difficulty in conceiving. Infertile ladies were recommended to drink large quantities of sage juice and refrain from sharing the conjugal bed for five days after their menstrual period. After this sage therapy they were told to 'live carnally with their husband'.

Sage has a high traditional reputation as a stimulant, one that was alleged to revive people almost at death's door. Unfortunately, this has not yet been supported by modern research.

Sage tea was widely used as a tonic and stimulant. An infusion is made in the usual way, allowing about one teaspoon of dried or fresh leaves to one cup of boiling water. This same mixture can be applied to the hair after shampooing to revive dark colours.

Asthma sufferers roll dried sage leaves up in cigarette papers and smoke them like tobacco to gain relief from their spasms. Sage leaves are still popularly chewed to whiten the teeth.

> Herbal Medicine <

Standard sage tea is recommended by herbalists for fevers, colds and all sore throats, both as a drink and a gargle. It is considered particularly valuable for ulcerated mouths.

Sage is recommended to nursing mothers to increase their milk yield and give tonic properties to the milk. Sage's tonic properties are appreciated herbally and used in medicine for depression. It is not generally given to highly strung, excitable patients.

Alternative medicine considers that sage is a fine aid to hair and scalp health, especially for those with darker hair. A strong infusion of sage leaves is made and drained, then rubbed into the scalp to stimulate the growth of hair and to get rid of dandruff.

> **Culinary Use** <

Sage has rather a strong taste, but if used sparingly it is a good addition to the herb shelf. It is superb with cheese, especially home-made varieties. Add a few chopped sage leaves to soya and other nuts when adding to savoury rice dishes. Sprinkle a few chopped fresh leaves over cooked spinach, onions, potatoes, aubergines or beetroot. Use sparingly with any rich meats or fish, such as goose, liver, pork, hare and beef. Sage is a good addition to herb butters.

> YOGURT <

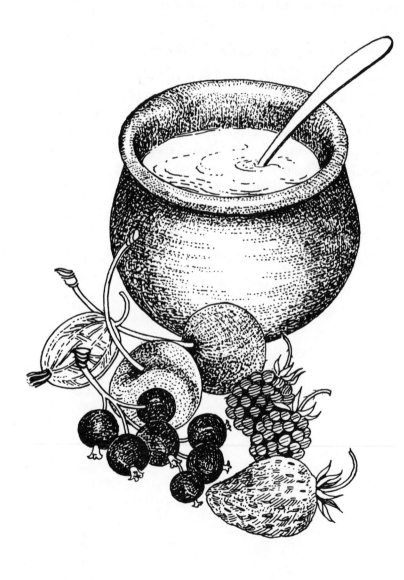

> Health <

Yogurt is such a well-known health food that it is a good idea to take a fresh look at it here. What exactly is yogurt and what does it do for us?

Yogurt originated among the nomadic tribes of Eastern Europe. Fresh milk turns sour when it is kept warm for a certain length of time, due to the action of organisms which convert some of the milk sugar – lactose – into lactic acid. Basically, a lactic fermentation takes place and the milk becomes what we know as yogurt.

In the Balkans and the Middle East they still make yogurt the traditional way by allowing warm milk to ferment. We can get the same results by adding yogurt culture to warm milk. This simple process is known technically as inoculation, and the organism which transforms milk into yogurt is *lactobacillus bulgaricus*. Commercial yogurt culture is made from this organism with the addition of *streptococcus thermophilus*.

Yogurt benefits our health in three main ways: it has a proven natural antibiotic quality; it can kill harmful bacteria in the intestine; it helps the body manufacture B vitamins.

Nobel prizewinner Ilya Metchnikoff first isolated the *lactobacillus bulgaricus* organism at the Pasteur Institute in Paris at the beginning of the century. Metchnikoff had been very impressed by the long life and vigour of Bulgarian peasants and other Balkan peoples who ate yogurt daily and drank large quantities of lactic acid milks.

'They are as strong as a root,' wrote Metchnikoff, and he devoted years of laboratory research to find out why.

The Nobel prizewinner had already come to the conclusion that much of the body's health is dependent on the health of the large intestine. In his research he found that yogurt produced friendly bacteria which killed disease bacteria in the large intestine.

Certain microbes hinder the putrefaction of milk. These are, in particular, the microbes that sour milk – that is, cause the formation of lactic acid – and which are antagonistic to the microbes of putrefaction. The lactic acid microbes hinder the multiplication of the organisms of putrefaction.

Metchnikoff published his findings in *The Prolongation of Life* in 1908, and caused waves of interest in yogurt throughout the entire world.

Research in the U.S.A. in the 1960s and 70s confirmed these early findings.

Dr Harry Seneca, writing in the *Journal of the American Geriatrics Association*, commented:

Yogurt contains some antibiotic principle which reaches its peak in 48 hours of growth and then gradually disappears over the next few weeks. All types of pathogenic bacteria and protozoa (harmful germs) are killed within five hours.

Further tests by Dr Seneca at Columbia University in the U.S.A. showed that when yogurt was eaten over a long period (a matter of months, regularly) no other bacteria except friendly yogurt bacteria appeared in the stools.

Yogurt's ability to kill germs was also noted by Dr David B. Sabine of the U.S. Vitamin and Pharmaceutical Corporation. Under controlled conditions, Dr Sabine grew harmful bacteria such as *staphylococcus* and *E. coli*. He added *lactobacillus* and *acidophilus* bacteria and observed that the harmful bacteria began gradually to disappear.

Yogurt's friendly bacteria have also been shown to help the intestinal flora manufacture the whole group of B vitamins. Powerful modern drugs, such as antibiotics, are known to kill off certain valuable intestinal flora. Long use of antibiotics can lead to B vitamin deficiencies, with symptoms of fatigue, depression, irritability and dry, cracked skin. For this reason, many nutritionally aware doctors now recommend natural yogurt to be taken at the same time as the medicine.

Throughout the East and in Greece, Bulgaria and Turkey a wide variety of cultured drinks are enjoyed as a daily beverage. These include *kefir*, known as the drink of the Prophet in Islamic countries; *koumiss* (fermented mare's milk); *ropa* (Finland); *gooddu* (Sardinia); *skuta* (Chile); *skyr* (Iceland); *chass* (India); and buttermilk, the traditional folk remedy of the American frontier, which certainly deserves to grace any list of popular lactic acid drinks.

People who are allergic to milk should try goats' milk yogurt, which they may well tolerate. Those with problem digestions might find that *kefir* or one of the other drinks would suit a delicate stomach better and still provide the excellent benefit of the lactic milk family.

> **Constituents** <

Yogurt contains calcium, iron, vitamin A, vitamin B1, niacin, a trace of vitamin C and linoleic acid, phosphorus and potassium.

> **History** <

According to an ancient tradition, an angel revealed to the prophet Abraham the method of making yogurt. The Bible tells us that Abraham lived to the age of 175 and fathered a child when he was 100, so this may well have planted the idea in the collective subconscious that yogurt is associated with longevity and fertility.

Galen, the Greek physician of the second century, advised his patients that yogurt had a beneficial and purifying effect on the whole system and was particularly good for bilious complaints. In the seventh century a treatise was published in Damascus called *The Great Explanation of the Power of the Elements*, in which yogurt was described as 'soothing, refreshing, regulating the intestinal tract and strengthening the stomach'.

Yogurt was known and valued in ancient or Eastern cultures long before it found a niche in the West.

In French popular history a story is told of how the aged, ailing Emperor François I ordered his doctors to find a medicine which could return some of his youthful vigour. The court physicians tried and failed miserably; learned doctors throughout the land sent secret potions and remedies. Nothing helped. Then, one doctor remembered he had heard of a secret formula in Constantinople which had a reputation for prolonging youth and vigour. A doctor from Constantinople was sent for immediately and he travelled to France on foot, driving his own flocks of sheep and carrying in his pocket precious yogurt culture.

The yogurt so transformed the Emperor François that it became known in France as *lait de la vie eternelle* – or milk of long life.

> **Folk Use** <

Throughout the Balkan countries people regularly take yogurt and cultured milk drinks, not only for longevity, but to ensure a healthy old age.

In Armenia and Georgia yogurt and *kefir* are used as a medicine to treat tuberculosis and typhoid. Researchers have found that there is a far lower incidence of diarrhoea among Russian babies because the mothers wean them on *kefir* or yogurt instead of whole milk.

Fermented milk products are widely used in Balkan folk medicine against diseases such as pneumonia, dysentery, and less serious complaints such as sore throats and laryngitis.

Bulgarian people use yogurt and lactic milk very much as tropical people use papaya, in short, as a complete medicine chest. Diarrhoea or any bowel disorders, gastritis, gout, constipation, fatigue, liver or kidney complaints and nervous disorders are all treated with lactic milk medicines.

In Bulgaria, where women are renowned for the beauty of

their complexions, yogurt is widely used as a skin lotion. Those with oily skins apply natural yogurt as a thick mask and leave it for at least an hour before rinsing off with warm water. Drier skins are treated to a combination of yogurt, lanolin and olive oil. Bulgarians make a most effective hair conditioner by mixing yogurt with eggs and a drop of olive oil. This is rubbed well into the scalp and left for about an hour before shampooing.

> **Herbal Medicine** <

Alternative medical practitioners believe that in some cases yogurt can be indigestible since it breaks into lumps during the digestive process. *Kefir*, on the other hand, breaks up into tiny particles and is to be preferred for those with acid stomachs, dyspepsia, or during 'irritated' conditions such as gastritis or colitis.

Normally, natural yogurt is highly recommended as part of a balanced diet. It is prescribed as a medicine during times of stress and when there is evidence of non-absorption of vitamins and minerals.

> **Culinary Use** <

If you buy commercial yogurt a few facts are worth knowing. Fat-free yogurt contains less than 0.5 per cent milk fat. Low fat yogurt contains no more than 1.5 per cent milk fat. Whole fruit or real fruit yogurt contains whole fruit in a sugar syrup. Fruit flavoured yogurt merely has a fruit juice syrup added.

Always buy yogurt from a refrigerated cabinet and see that the date stamp on the lid has not expired. If a thickening agent or colour additive has been included, it should be shown in the list of ingredients.

Naturopaths and all alternative medicine practitioners greatly prefer natural, plain yogurt. This is very easy to make at home and quite a bit cheaper than the commercial product.

All you need to do is to bring milk to the warm temperature

of 43°C. (110°F.) – which is just above body temperature. It should feel comfortable if you test it with a clean finger. Sterilized or long life milk will give the best results. Fresh pasteurized milk may be used, but must be boiled first, then covered and allowed to cool down to the required 43°C. (110°F.) temperature. A common cause of failure when making yogurt is using fresh milk and not boiling it first, because animals are often given antibiotics which appear in the milk and 'fight' the yogurt bacteria.

If you regularly make large amounts of yogurt it is well worth investing in a special electric yogurt-making kit which stays at the correct temperature. However, a pre-warmed wide-necked vacuum flask can be just as effective. Whatever you use, make sure it is perfectly clean and make the yogurt in this way:-

1. Pour a litre of milk into a saucepan and heat to 43°C. (110°F.). Use the finger test or a thermometer to check the temperature.

2. Add two tablespoons of fresh natural yogurt and mix well, or add a packet of dried yogurt culture.

3. Pour the milk into the clean vacuum flask or yogurt kit container. Close securely and leave undisturbed for eight to ten hours to set.

4. Put the yogurt in a covered container in the refrigerator until required for use.

Skimmed milk, soya bean milk, goats' milk or buttermilk may all be used to make yogurt. A thicker, creamier yogurt can be made by adding skimmed milk powder to the mixture in the beginning. Allow about one level tablespoon to each 568 ml. Many people prefer the taste of this fortified version.

In cooking, the slightly acidic flavour of yogurt enhances many dishes. It can be delicious added to casseroles, but never try to boil or overheat it because it will separate. A delicious country casserole is made with cider, pork, onions, celery, mushrooms and a carton of natural yogurt. Mix the other ingredients and casserole them in the usual way for about one and a half hours or until the meat is tender. Mix the yogurt with a little of the hot liquid, return to the pan and reheat without boiling. Adjust the seasoning before serving.

Yogurt can be added to cheese sauces after they have been heated and mixed, just before serving. A delicious yogurt sauce is made with one cup of yogurt, two tablespoons of lemon juice or cider vinegar, one teaspoon of Worcester sauce, one quarter teaspoon of dry mustard, two tablespoons each of well grated onion, parsley and zest of a lemon, and sprinkle of cayenne pepper. Mix well and serve with cold vegetables, fish or cold meats. As it is, plain natural yogurt is a great addition to salads. Thinly sliced cucumber in yogurt is a popular Middle Eastern and Indian dish, served either as a starter or as part of a salad meal. Crunchy eating apples and celery are also good diced and mixed in yogurt.

A good salad dressing can be made with natural yogurt mixed with salt, pepper, chopped chives and lemon juice. This dressing goes particularly well with apple, celery or walnut salads, especially Waldorf salad.

Delicious instant desserts can be made with yogurt. Blend equal amounts of natural yogurt and fruit purée together for a quick fruit fool. Put a layer of stewed fruit or fruit salad, then a layer of yogurt, and top it with crunchy granola-type cereal or chopped nuts just before serving, for a superb dessert.

> INDEX <

Index

Index

Index

Pregnancy, 108, 192: diet during, 35, 47, 93, 143, 169; toxaemia of, 93
Prostate gland, 47
Protein drinks, high, 41
Pruritus, 151
Psoriasis, 147
Puberty, 39, 192

Raspberry, 39, 58
Rasputin, 107
Red currant, 46
Rejuvenator, 102, 108, 167
Renwick, Sir James, 181
Rheumatism, 108, 135: chronic, 126; folk remedies for, 10, 22, 36, 66, 67, 81, 82, 97, 125, 126, 158, 186; herb tea recommended for, 37, 39; herbal treatment for, 68, 81, 87, 98, 173, 180; poultice for, 120, 137, 160
Rice water, 43
Ringworm, 172
Rooibosch tea, 40
Rosehip syrup, 43
Royal jelly, *see* Honey
Rudge, Dr Christopher, 165
'Run-down feeling', *see* Debility
Rutin, 39

Sabine, Dr David B., 196
Safflower oil, 41
Sage, 39, 68, 115, **191-3**: juice, 192; tea, 191
Salt-free diet, 122
Sarsaparilla, 14, 39
Sauerkraut, 65, 71, 91, 127: antibiotic properties of, 68; prevention against scurvy, 66
Scars, 114
Sciatica, 98, 126, 135, 186
Scurf, *see* Dandruff
Scurvy, 36, 47, 66, 165, 184, 186
Sedative, natural, 103, 114, 130, 131
Seneca, Dr H., 196
Senna pods, 39
Sexual activity, 131, 132; debility, 31, 102; virility, 105, 107
Shakers, 52, 108
Shallots, 161
Shaternikov, Professor V. A., 10

Shultes, Professor Richard Evan, 14
Shrive, Dr William, 64
Sight, poor, 66
Sinusitis, 119, 121
Skin: beautifier, 114, 115; care of, 142; cleanser, 158; conditioner, 144, 147, 186; herbal treatment for, 187; lotion, 144, 199; oily, 60; stimulant, 141; toner, 179
Skin complaints, 81
Slimming, 26, 34, 59, 78, 79, 85, 182: bran and, 59; food to avoid during, 36; hunger pangs of, 35, 79, 89; oil-free diet, effect of, 147 (*see also* Diet, Weight loss)
Smörgåsbord, 76
Soap substitute, 60
Sores, 108, 166
Sore throats, 46, 47, 48: bromelin and, 177; folk remedies for, 47, 67, 97, 191; gargle for, 36, 46, 47, 52, 53, 67, 115, 166, 178, 192; herbal treatment for, 39, 48, 159, 179, 192
Soups, 31, 70, 99, 133, 145, 151
Spring cleanser, traditional folk, 11, 22, 29, 86, 98, 126, 129
St George, George, *Russian Folk Medicine*, 107
Stamina, 104
Sterility, 102
Stimulant, natural, 103, 104, 108, 136, 144, 158, 191, 192
Stings, 172
Stomach: complaints of, 36, 144; infections of, 68, 127
Strawberry, 58
Stress, 109: adapting to, 103; herb tea recommended for, 38
Strokes, 22
Succory, *see* Chicory
Sunburn, 151, 186
Sunflower oil, 41, 152
Sweet cicely, 39

Tan, instant, 151
Tapeworm, 98
Tea, *see* Herb tea, and individual names
Teeth, whitener, 192

Index

Temperature, *see* Fever
Throats: ulcerated, 115; relaxed, 191 (*see also* Sore throats)
Thurber, James, *Alarms and Diversions*, 14
Thyme, 39
Tiredness, *see* Fatigue, Exhaustion
Tonic: natural, 34, 51, 53, 78, 79, 81, 82, 87, 98, 102, 108, 192; nerve, 52, 81, 144; spring, 120 (*see also* Spring cleanser)
Tonsillitis, 158, 191
Tranquillizer, natural, 90, 130
Tuberculosis, 97, 179, 198
Turner, William, 171
Turnip, 58
Typhoid, 198

U.S. Department of Agriculture, 10, 57
U.S. Pharmacopoeia, 191
U.S. Senate Select Committee, 11
Ulcers, stomach: food recommended for, 144; herb tea recommended for, 38; peptic, 65, 68, 179; treatment by cabbage extracts, 10, 65, 68
Underweight, 38
Urinary disorders, 124, 159: drink recommended for, 41, 43, 48
Urine, retention of, 48

Varicose veins, 57
Vegetable oil, 51, 148, 152

Vermifuge, 98 (*see also* Parasites)
Vichy water, *see* Mineral waters
Virility, 102: loss of, 39, 81, 104 (*see also* Sexual activity)
Virus 94: protection against, 22
Vitality, 96, 115; lack of, 37, 38 (*see also* Energy)
Vitamin A, food rich in, 27, 170
Vitamin B: food rich in, 142; deficiencies of, 196; manufacture in the body of, 195
Vitamin C, food rich in, 35, 43, 46, 51, 165, 170
Vitamin E, food rich in, 130

Warts, 166, 167
Water retention, 169
Weight loss, 26 (*see also* Slimming, Diet)
Wheat, bread, 56, 58, 60, 61
Whooping cough, 96, 97, 98
Williams, Dr Roger, 64
Wine, medicated, 44
Wind, *see* Flatulence
Worms, *see* Parasites
Wounds, 68, 126, 165, 166
Wrinkles, 115: prevention of, 158

Yeast, 59
Yogurt, 41, 98, **195–201**: anti-bacteria agents of, 195, 196; home-made, 200; salad dressing, 201

208